Your Stomach

Your Stomach

*What Is Really Making You Miserable
and What To Do About It*

Jonathan V. Wright, M.D.

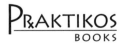

DISCLAIMER

Ideas and information in this book are based upon the experience and training of the author and the scientific information currently available. The suggestions in this book are definitely not meant to be a substitute for careful medical evaluation and treatment by a qualified, licensed health professional. The author and publisher do not recommend changing or adding medication or supplements without consulting your personal physician. They specifically disclaim any liability arising directly or indirectly from the use of this book.

Praktikos Books
P.O. Box 118
Mount Jackson, VA 22842
888.542.9467   info@praktikosbooks.com

Praktikos Books are produced in alliance with Axios Press.

Distributed by National Book Network.

Library of Congress Cataloging-in-Publication Data

Wright, Jonathan V.
    Your stomach : what is really making you miserable and what to do about it / Jonathan V. Wright.
        p.   cm.
    Includes bibliographical references and index.
    ISBN 978-1-60766-000-2 (alk. paper)

    1. Gastroesophageal reflux—Popular works. 2. Gastric acid—Popular works. 3. Heartburn—Popular works. 4. Antacids—Side effects—Popular works. I. Title.

RC815.7.W75 2009
616.3′24—dc22

2009011166

Contents

Your Stomach

A GREENWICH, CONNECTICUT money manager in his early 50s has made a vast fortune. He is being interviewed by *Vanity Fair* magazine about the 30,000-square foot home he is building. As the interview proceeds, the money manager pops a powerful antacid pill and sips from a glass of lactose-free skim milk.

One wonders: Will the manager enjoy his new mansion (or anything else) if his stomach is always hurting? If he could choose between the mansion and a sound stomach, wouldn't he choose a sound stomach? Wouldn't anybody?

A Very Widespread Problem

It is not just rich people who are popping antacids continually, who are literally afraid to eat, and who dread going to bed after eating dinner. Evidence suggests that a majority of adult Americans have stomach problems to one degree or another; many of them lead lives of utter misery.

An estimated 40–44% of adult Americans suffer from a particular stomach malady called acid reflux. This is acid backing up the throat from the stomach, and is commonly referred to as "heartburn."[1] Chronic acid reflux may be diagnosed as gastro-esophageal reflux disease (GERD). GERD in turn is associated with throat cancer, which is America's fastest growing malignancy, up six fold over the past two decades.*[2]

---

* 16,470 Americans are expected to be diagnosed with throat cancer in 2008, with only one in five expected to survive over five years. Many more patients have pre-cancerous throat lesions and many more have "Barrett's esophagus," which can lead to pre-cancerous lesions. Pre-cancerous lesions are often "burned" off the throat, or in some cases the esophagus is surgically removed. A Georgetown University study is currently looking at "burning" throats before they become pre-cancerous.

A research study suggests that the risk of developing Barrett's can be substantially (65%) reduced by eating a diet high in fruits,

A Medical Mistake?

The irony in all this is that these millions of sufferers may be the victims of a medical mistake. Medical mistakes are not uncommon in history. George Washington seems to have been bled to death by his doctors, and there are many other famous cases. But rarely in history has a medical mistake affected so many millions of people, which appears to be the case today with stomach remedies.

We Need Stomach Acid

The basic misconception is that acid, stomach acid, too much stomach acid, is causing the stomach distress and heartburn. The solution is, therefore, to reduce or even eliminate the acid by taking antacids. What this fails to recognize is that the stomach is designed to hold very strong acid.

We need the acid to break down and digest our food,[5] or to convert food from one form to

---

vegetables, and non-fried fish.[3] Research also suggests that the risk is increased by a high consumption of soft drinks.[4]

another. For example, iron in food is converted from a non-absorbable to an absorbable form. This is vital because we need iron to live. In addition, the presence of strong acid triggers the release of enzymes and hormones that we absolutely need to complete the digestion process.[6]

If we do not have enough acid, we are likely to experience the symptoms of:

- Stomach or esophageal pain (heartburn or reflux from half digested food backing up the throat).

- Bloating, belching, often constipation.
- "Food just sits in the stomach."[7]

And for women:

- "My fingernails break and crack no matter what I do."

Or:

- "My hair just keeps on thinning and falling out."[8]

Stomach Acid Declines with Age

Most people do not know that stomach acid tends to decline with age.[9] Young people on average have lots of stomach acid. Do they develop stomach problems? Not usually.

Infants of course do tend to throw up food, but this is usually outgrown and frequently stops once milk and dairy products are eliminated. Some doctors have begun to give infants and children antacids[10] with predictable results. The children develop more serious stomach problems and may not outgrow them.[11]

It is older people who report the most stomach trouble. When they do, most doctors do not check the actual level of stomach acid produced in the patient's stomach. Tests are often made of acid levels in the throat. Even when endoscopes are used to check the interior stomach surface for ulcers, stomach acid levels are not generally tested.[12]

When doctors have performed actual stomach acid tests in grown adults, they have often been surprised to find so little acid.[13] If acid has fallen to low levels, and the patient is having stomach trouble, how can it make sense to eliminate what little acid is left?

What Really Causes Heartburn

But, you may respond: When acid reflux comes up the throat, it burns, often painfully. Doesn't that mean there is too much acid in the stomach? Also, what about a "sour" feeling in the stomach? Isn't that further proof that there is too much acid?

The answer in both cases is no. Partly digested food is not supposed to back up the throat. Once food has passed into the stomach, a valve at the top of the stomach should hold it back.[14] There are cases in which what is called a hiatal hernia may interfere with the normal valve mechanism, but this is true only for a small minority of cases, which will require surgery.

The throat is not made for acid.[15] Even a little acid there will produce that unpleasant burning sensation. The stomach by contrast is made for acid. Its thick lining protects it. An amount of acid that causes intense distress in the throat is absolutely normal in the stomach.[16]

The challenge for the great majority of refluxers who do not have a hiatal hernia is to keep the acid in the stomach where it belongs. This means keeping the upper stomach valve closed.[17] If the valve functions properly, what is meant to be in the stomach will stay there. And we will neither experience reflux in our throat nor a more general sour feeling.

Why would the valve function improperly? In some cases, it could be caused by:[18]

- Food allergies and sensitivities,
- Caffeine,
- Alcohol,
- Nicotine.

But as we shall see, there is another possible explanation for reflux.

What Else Might Cause Acid to Back Up Into the Throat?

Some medical researchers have suggested that there is a problem of too much acid in the stomach.[19] But most of the research is clear: dampening stomach acid does not help the valve perform better.[20]

If medical research does not support the idea that too much acid causes the valve to malfunction, why use antacids?

The usual argument goes as follows: Yes, antacids won't help the malfunctioning valve. But since the valve is malfunctioning, since partly digested food is backing up into the throat, let's make that food less acidic, less painful for the throat. The heartburn will still happen, but there will be less discomfort, pain, or damage for the throat.

What do opponents of using antacids say to that? They say that antacids often make the heartburn worse. They are not entirely sure why. One guess is that the proper functioning of the valve below the throat actually requires a good deal of acid in the stomach.[21]

Why Antacids Might Make the Situation Worse

The basic idea here is that the stomach begins to fill with acid as we eat. The valve remains open so that food can pass into the stomach. After we have eaten, the acid level rises further to complete digestion. Once the acid reaches a certain level, the stomach sends a signal to close the valve. If acid does not rise to the required level, no signal is given and the valve remains open or partly open. Could the stomach signal the rest of the body to close the valve?

The intestinal tract, including the stomach, is lined with "communication" cells that are similar to the cells in our brain. So the idea that the stomach signals the body to close the valve when stomach acid levels rise is perfectly possible. Even so, it remains a guess. It has not yet been scientifically proven.[22]

What if this idea is correct? What would we expect to happen if we try to reduce the symptoms of the heartburn by taking antacids? That is, what would we expect to happen if we reduce stomach acidity?

The result will be less stomach acid. And, in that case, the stomach will never signal the body to close the valve. The acid that backs into the throat may be weaker but there will be more of it. The problem gets worse, not better.

Of course, heartburn is not the only stomach problem afflicting people. What about stomach pain, which is usually associated with gas? This gas may take the form of bloating. In that case, the sufferer has no doubt that the problem is gas.

Sometimes the gas attack is stealthy. One feels pain, either a sharp or a dull pain, but not bloated. The pain may be truly intense.

The sufferer may even mistake this intense pain for a heart attack.[23] Off he or she goes to the emergency room of the hospital, where one waits and waits and waits, only—in the end—to be given an antacid.

Why an antacid in this case? Because an antacid, often combined with a gas-absorbing chemical, will provide temporary relief. The pain will subside.

Unfortunately, sooner or later, the pain will likely return. And the occurrences may become more frequent. In many cases, eating any food at all will bring on an attack. One then eats, takes an antacid, eats, takes an antacid. Next, one takes a strong, prescription antacid that shuts down most acid production all day. But the stomach is still not right. It often gets worse and worse as time passes.

Why Do Antacids Appear to Help—At Least Temporarily?

What is happening here? Why does the antacid provide temporary relief of symptoms but not a cure? Why does the problem, indeed, often get worse?

Neither the proponents nor the opponents of antacids know for sure. Given the huge sales of antacids, it is surprising that there has not been more scientific research designed to provide answers. We are still at the stage of guessing.

The proponents of antacids guess that there is too much acid in the stomach for optimal digestion and this contributes to gas formation. The problem with this guess is that, as we have seen, acid production declines with age and many stomach sufferers, when tested for acid production, turn out to be very low in acid.

Moreover, a search of major medical databases containing over 16,000 scientific research articles on stomach ailments reveals no evidence whatsoever that stomach acid is the source of the problem. This is true whether the specific stomach complaint is reflux, general stomach pain, or ulcers.

What Is Really Happening?

Opponents of antacids guess that a lack of acid prevents normal digestion. The food then begins to ferment. Fermentation is certainly better than nothing. Without fermentation, food would not be broken down, would just remain where it is, blocking the system. Supporting the "fermentation idea" are the results of a single medical experiment performed over 100 years ago. The investigating physician used a tube to suck out stomach contents from heartburn sufferers, and found acetic and butyric acids, known products of bacterial fermentation.[24]

But fermentation is not the optimal approach. One of its many disadvantages is the production of excess gas.[25] There are also reasons to doubt that we get as much nutrition from food that is not digested in the normal way. We may be eating enough, but nutritionally starving ourselves.

Why antacids provide temporary relief from fermenting food in the stomach is also a mystery. It may be that antacids, by further reducing stomach acid levels, tend to interrupt the fermentation process. If so, the food will ferment at a slower pace, or may stop fermenting for awhile and then recommence.

This will reduce the pain temporarily, but not solve the problem. The patient's stomach will still not feel "right." When more food is consumed, the pain will start up again.

Doesn't Everybody "Know" that Antacids are the Stomach Medicine of Choice?

Good question. Is it really possible that antacids harm us? Everyone "knows" that antacids are the best stomach medicine. But consider, for a moment, how everyone has come to "know" this. Isn't it primarily through advertising? Patent medicine companies (generally known as "pharmaceutical" or "drug" companies) have become rich by advertising antacids. Until the arrival of statins (to reduce cholesterol), they were the best selling patent medicines (pharmaceutical drugs) of all time.[26] They are still the number two seller. Consider these facts:

■ Drug companies currently sell over $20 billion worth of antacids a year.[27] This is not including over-the-counter antacids.
■ Two patent medicines sold by the drug company AstraZeneca, Prilosec, and Nexium, currently have $6.55 billion in sales. This is almost 25% of AstraZeneca's total revenues.[28]

- Drug companies spend an estimated $30 to $60 billion a year on advertising.[29] Much of this advertises antacids.

What Drug Companies Actually Say

If you listen carefully to the antacid ads on TV or read them in magazines, they do not offer scientific evidence that too much acid causes stomach problems. For the most part, they do not even make the claim.[30] They simply describe the pain and show someone getting relief with their product.

Drug companies provide more information about antacids on websites and on package inserts. What do we find there?

The Prilosec website[31] says that heartburn can be triggered by a variety of factors: what you eat or drink, an unrelated illness, the way you live. These triggers in turn can lead to: a relaxed LES (lower esophageal valve), more acid production, pressure on the stomach, or a more sensitive esophagus (throat). None of this, of course, claims that stomach acid causes heartburn.

This website acknowledges that Prilosec works by "directly blocking many active acid pumps in the stomach." In the prescribing information for doctors,[32] we learn that up to 90% of stomach acid may be eliminated for twenty-four hours or longer.

The website goes on to say that "Your stomach still produces enough acid to digest the food you eat," but offers no scientific proof that this is true. As we shall see later, this is an unsupported claim. There are reasons to believe that it is false.

The National Heartburn Alliance makes the same claim: that even the strongest antacids do not prevent "normal digestion."[33] But the Alliance is drug company funded.

More importantly, the Mayo Clinic, a widely respected bastion of conventional medicine, has said the same in its newsletter:

> Although most antacids can be quite effective at reducing (neutralizing) acid in your stomach, even the most potent acid-reducing drugs have no discernible effect on the digestive process.[34]

Unfortunately the Mayo Clinic did not cite any sources. For a claim that defies common sense (by arguing that we don't need the acid that nature put in our bodies), we should expect to see many scientific studies, not only of the immediate consequences of suppressing acid, but of the long-term consequences as well.

www.gerd.com (sponsored by AstraZeneca, the drug company which makes the powerful and popular antacid Nexium) does state that:

> The short- and long-term safety of PPI's (proton pump inhibitors such as Prilosec and Nexium) has been confirmed in many large studies.

In making this statement, it cites a research study by P. N. Maton.[35]

What does Dr. Maton actually say? The abstract of Dr. Maton's article says, among other things, that: "The efficacy [effectiveness] of antacids . . . has not been proven definitively in clinical trials." Nor does the article demonstrate that strong antacids are safe for long-term use. Indeed, as we shall see, there are many studies suggesting the opposite. Even the package inserts for Prilosec and Nexium say that these patent medicines are for short-term use.[36]

Don't Many Doctors Agree with the Drug Companies?

Don't most doctors agree with the drug companies? Don't they prescribe Prilosec and other strong antacids? Don't they often prescribe them for the short and long term? The answer, unfortunately, is yes. Most doctors do assume that too much stomach acid, not too little, is causing their patients' heartburn and other stomach troubles.

Why is this? In the first place, the doctors see the same ads you do. They read studies financed by the drug companies. Some of their education, and in many cases most of their continuing education, is financed by the drug companies.[37]

Doesn't the Government Support the Use of Antacids?

The prescription antacids themselves are approved by the US Food and Drug Administration (FDA). Many FDA panelists are hired by the drug companies.[38] Congress recently passed legislation to reduce this abuse but not eliminate it.[39] And a substantial portion of the FDA's budget is paid for by the drug companies.[40]

Does this mean that scientific research on the benefits of stomach acid and the potential harm of antacids will never be acknowledged or circulated within the mainstream medical community? No. But it does mean that it may take longer to change minds and change medical practice than it should.

Why Antacids May Be Bad for Your Bones

If the critics of antacids are right, this almost universal stomach medicine is making stomachs perform worse, not better. It is causing untold suffering and misery among stomach sufferers. But that is not the end of the story, far from it.

Common sense tells us that nature put acid in the stomach for a reason: to help us digest food. If we don't digest our food properly, we will be malnourished,[41] and malnourishment can in turn lead to a host of other problems.

If this common sense view is correct, the use of powerful antacids should eventually lead to trouble outside the stomach. A landmark research study published in the *Journal of the American Medical Association* in 2006 provided strong evidence that the long-term use of powerful antacids is associated with:

- hip fracture,[42] which may itself be a symptom of weak bones;[43] or
- osteoporosis.[44]

Although the study focused on hip fracture, the likelihood is that other bones are being weakened by antacids as well. Why would this be the case?

A number of studies have found that stomach acid is very important for the absorption of the mineral calcium.[45] We know that calcium is important for bones. But there are probably many other minerals and factors involved, all of which may depend to some degree on stomach acid for absorption.[46]

Please also keep in mind that calcium in the body is a de-acidifying mineral. It reduces acidity in the body. But stomach acid helps get it in the body in the first place.

So Acidity in the Stomach and Acidity in the Rest of the Body are Two Separate Issues?

That is correct. Even if testing of blood or saliva suggests that your body is too acidic, it does not follow that you need to reduce stomach acid. The reverse may be true.

You may have seen advertisements selling pills or powders to "deacidify your body." Often the pills or powders are antacids that you are told to eat or drink, which means they will pass through your stomach.

Do not be misled by these ads. Your stomach is designed for a high level of acid. The rest of your body is not. It is perfectly true that your body must maintain the right degree of overall acidity for optimum health. But it does not follow that you should, therefore, further lower the acidity of your stomach.

Conclusion: Don't listen to those who vilify acid, particularly stomach acid. What the body needs is acid in the right balance, and especially in the right places, especially in the stomach—that is what nature intended.

Other Medical Conditions Associated with Low Stomach Acid

In addition to hip fracture, continued use of patent medicines which cause low—or no—stomach acid has been associated with other medical conditions such as:

- clostridial bowel infections[47]
- macular degeneration[48]
- dementia[49]
- depletion of vitamin C[50]
- pneumonia[51]

Even the most conventional medical textbook agrees that stomach acid is in the stomach for a good reason. One role of acid is to help digest food, especially proteins and minerals. The acid does this directly, by breaking down or converting food, but also indirectly, by triggering the release of important enzymes and, perhaps, by triggering other events (such as closing the LES valve that protects the throat).

Digestion, however, is still not the whole story. Conventional medical textbooks also agree that stomach acid is the "acid barrier" protecting the body from invading and unwanted microorganisms such as bacteria and fungi.[52] These microorganisms commonly enter our body through the mouth or nose but meet their doom in the acid environment of the stomach. In addition to killing many disease-causing microorganisms, acid from our stomachs helps maintain normal "friendly" microorganisms in the twenty or more feet of our intestines, and discourage the growth of "unfriendly" microorganisms. Because acid protects us, one would expect that antacids would lower our defenses against infection. This assumption needs more research. But in addition to the link between antacids and pneumonia mentioned above, some studies have indicated a link between antacids and both bacterial overgrowth[53] and fungal infections such as *Candida albicans*.[54] This overgrowth has also been linked to bile reflux and esophageal cancer.[55]

Decades ago, during a cholera epidemic, physicians investigated why part of the people in a village would get the sometimes fatal diarrheal disease, but another part did not. They reported that the people who avoided cholera had much stronger stomach acid than those who came down with the disease.[56] The physicians concluded that stronger stomach acid kills the cholera bacteria before it causes disease further down the intestines.

Antacids and Stomach Ulcers

There may also be a link between antacids and stomach ulcers. If so, this is ironic, since antacids are used as an adjunct therapy for ulcers.

Stomach ulcers are usually described as "holes" in the stomach lining. They are often, but not always, associated with stomach pain and bloating.

For years, conventional medicine thought they were caused by diet or, especially, stress. In the early 1980s, two Australian doctors, Robin Warren and Barry James Marshall, argued that ulcers were instead caused by a bacterium, *Helicobacter pylori* (*H. pylori*). For years, conventional medicine rejected this idea, and the two pioneering doctors were ridiculed and subjected to personal abuse. Eventually, however, their bacterial theory prevailed.[57] Since then, *H. pylori* has also been linked to stomach cancer.[58]

The usual treatment for ulcers today is a round of antibiotics to kill the *H. pylori* bacteria combined with a strong antacid supposedly designed to help the stomach lining heal. The logic of this, however, is hard to understand.

H. pylori is killed by acid. It tends to bore into the stomach lining at least in part to escape acid. Reducing acid by antacid use would, logically, help the *H. pylori* survive the antibiotics.

Moreover, recent research has found that *H. pylori* actually causes the stomach to produce less acid.[59] This might help explain why *H. pylori* can cause stomach cancer, since the absence of stomach acid is a precondition for developing that type of cancer.[60]

In addition, various studies have shown natural treatments to be effective at healing ulcers without negative side effects. Mastic gum is often cited.[61] Cabbage juice has also been used.[62] Some clinicians recommend taking cayenne pepper[63] along with the cabbage juice, a combination that has been shown to eradicate *H. pylori* in seven to ten days.

Deglycyrrhizinated licorice (DGL) is supported by some research, but the evidence is less clear.[64] Note that regular licorice root can be toxic and licorice candy rarely contains real licorice.

Recent research has also suggested that virgin olive oil may kill *H. pylori*.[65] If so, olive leaf extract might be effective as well. Rhubarb or cranberry may be effective, too.[66] Why then would many doctors still use the antacids for ulcers? Perhaps because they are accustomed to using them, or because the drug company making the antacid has persuaded them to include antacids with the antibiotic.

Additional Medical Conditions that Might Be Indirectly Linked to Low Stomach Acid

These conditions may be related to deficient stomach acid, but probably not in a direct cause–effect relationship. Instead there may be a "third factor" causing both the disease and the low stomach acid. In some cases, this "third factor" may have a connection with food allergies or intolerances linked to substances such as gluten (found in wheat products) or eggs. The "third factor" may also be a higher degree of "genetic pre-disposition" in the same person to develop both low stomach acid and the associated disease.

Whatever its origin, if the low stomach acid goes undetected, it's a lot harder to treat the disease as multiple nutrients will not be absorbed well; and the body has a harder time fighting the disease without them. Some medical conditions that may be related in this way with deficient stomach acid are:

- Acne rosacea[67]
- Addison's disease[68]
- Allergies and allergic reactions[69]
- Celiac disease[70]
- Childhood asthma[71]
- Chronic autoimmune hepatitis[72]
- Diabetes (type I—Juvenile)[73]
- Eczema (severe)[74]
- Gallbladder disease[75]
- Graves' disease (hyperthyroid)[76]
- Lupus erythematosus[77]
- Multiple sclerosis[78]
- Myasthenia gravis[79]
- Pernicious anemia[80]
- Polymyalgia rheumatica[81]
- Raynaud's syndrome[82]
- Rheumatoid arthritis[83]
- Scleroderma[84]
- Sjögren's syndrome[85]
- Ulcerative colitis[86]
- Vitiligo[87]

Much more scientific research is needed to establish whether a provable link exists between these diseases and low stomach acid. But based on:

- Actual testing of stomach acid in thousands of "heartburn" sufferers since 1976 with a technique also used by major drug companies.
- The fact that the majority of these conditions are "HLA-linked" (HLA testing is a way of predicting risk of disease).
- My own clinical experience.

It appears that a link exists.

Side Effects of Prescription-Strength Antacids

Chronic diseases and infections associated or possibly associated with antacids might seem to be enough to worry about. But let's not forget that prescription-strength antacids are powerful patent medicines, and like all such drugs they come with worrying side effects.

To study the potential side effects, one need only review the package inserts. Some of the potential side effects mentioned for Prilosec and/or Nexium include:[88]

- Headache
- Diarrhea
- Upper respiratory tract infections
- Dizziness
- Constipation
- Back pain
- Depression
- Pancreatic inflammation
- Liver damage
- Allergic reaction, such as rash, hives, or unexplained swelling
- Loss of appetite
- Dry mouth
- Weight gain
- Muscle cramps
- Joint pain
- Insomnia
- Drowsiness
- Vertigo
- Hair loss

- Dry skin
- Blurred vision
- Tinnitus (ringing in the ears)
- Taste changes
- Dry eyes
- Urinary tract infections
- Anemia

On top of that, a study published in the *Journal of the American Medical Association* found that patients who suffer a heart attack nearly double the risk of having another if they are taking the widely used blood thinner Plavix together with a heartburn drug like Prilosec or Nexium, and are 25 percent more likely to die or be readmitted to a hospital. Because Plavix increases the risk of dangerous gastrointestinal bleeding, many doctors routinely give protein pump inhibitor drugs like Prilosec to patients on Plavix.[89]

The Case against Antacids

The case against antacids may be summed up as follows:

- They only offer short-term, symptomatic relief.
- They make the problem worse over the long term.
- Reducing stomach acid is a radical step, and may lead to a host of chronic diseases or infections, quite apart from the patent medicine's acknowledged side effects.

The Alternative Approach to Stomach Problems

If one accepts this argument, or accepts that it might be correct, the conclusion would be to avoid antacids, or at least use them with extreme caution, or only under rare circumstances.

Logically, the next question would be whether to treat a malfunctioning stomach with more acid rather than less. This question would be especially logical for older people with stomach complaints, given the studies showing a decline in stomach acid production with age.

There are folk remedies that take this approach. For example, apple cider vinegar is often found among folk remedies for stomach disorders.[90]

Some apple cider vinegars are much stronger than others. A popular brand of organic apple cider vinegar, Bragg, has a 5% acidity. That makes it less acidic than most commercial brands. It should also be noted that apple cider vinegar contains acetic acid, not the hydrochloric acid that the human stomach produces.

Hydrochloric acid capsules (which also contain pepsin, a protein-digesting enzyme made by the stomach) are available as supplements sold in health food stores. These are usually sold as Betaine HCL with pepsin. No one, of course, should use acid except with the advice and under the care of a licensed doctor.

It is generally unrecognized that restoring stomach acid (HCL-pepsin) to more youthful levels is also a powerful and all-natural *anti-aging* treatment. If we restore our digestive system with HCL, we are again able to benefit

from all the nutrition in our food, so that our
bodies receive a better flow of:

- Essential amino acids. These are essential not only for strong muscles, but also
  are the precursors of the large majority of
  our brain's messenger molecules, called
  "neurotransmitters."

- Minerals. We'll take up more calcium
  and keep our bones much healthier.
  We'll take up more iron—HCL is essential for absorption of this important
  mineral, which is key to making enough
  hemoglobin to oxygenate our tissues.
  Many other minerals are also at least
  partially dependent on normal levels of
  HCL-pepsin to be absorbed.

- Folate (also called "folic acid"). One of the
  "top two" vitamin deficiencies, folate is
  very important to mental health in older
  individuals, and has been found to lower
  risk of several cancers.

- Absorption of adequate amounts of vitamins A, D, E, K, and essential fatty acids
  (EFA) may be indirectly compromised if

there's not enough HCL produced by the stomach to properly activate the entire "digestive cascade."

- Vitamin C production. No one knows why, but one study shows lower levels of vitamin C in individuals who took acid blockers for a longer period of time.[91]

- Vitamin B12 absorption may be especially problematic, as "missing stomach acid" isn't the only problem here, but also the absence of another absorption molecule not made well if the stomach lining is too atrophied. Vitamin B12 absorption should be discussed with a physician skilled and knowledgeable about these topics.

As you've read, many, many nutrients may not be properly digested and absorbed if your stomach acid is too low. Without these important "repair materials," health will decline more rapidly! That's why restoring more normal digestion with HCL-pepsin is truly part of an *anti-aging* program.

An *integrative* doctor, one who combines the use of supplements and natural remedies with patent medicines, if necessary, can measure the patient's stomach acid to see if a deficiency exists. This involves swallowing a monitor which is then retrieved (not a pleasant experience but no worse—many say much less bad—than an invasive endo- or gastroscope).

If acid is low, the doctor will then decide whether acid supplementation with meals is indicated, and if so, the best way to do it. The doctor may suggest other natural remedies as well. We have already discussed some natural ways to control an *H. pylori* infection. Some research suggests that d-Limonene, an orange peel extract, may help with the symptoms of heartburn.[92]

If acid is normal (in my experience, this would be true for only a minority of those suffering from "heartburn" or GERD), the physician will usually recommend testing for food allergies and sensitivities, or supplements which strengthen the function of the valve which separates the esophagus from the stomach, or other natural means which relieve heartburn but don't interfere with normal digestion.

Among these natural means may be supplementing melatonin, the natural "sleep" hormone which also declines with age. Recent "controlled" research compared melatonin to omeprazole, one of the most widely sold acid blockers, in their ability to eliminate heartburn. After 7 days of use, 100% of 176 individuals using 6 milligrams of melatonin after dinner (along with small amounts of L-trypotophan, L-methionine, vitamin B6, vitamin B12, folic acid, and betaine) had symptom relief, and by forty days had complete relief of heartburn. In the omeprazole group (175 individuals), 65.7% had symptom relief after nine days; the remainder (34.3%) had persistent symptoms for the entire forty days.

After the forty days, the 34.3% not relieved of symptoms by omeprazole were all given the melatonin and other nutrients. All of these individuals had relief of their heartburn, too. The melatonin with other nutrients clearly outperformed the omeprazole, and very importantly, melatonin does not interfere with normal digestion.[93]

In a single-case report, the physician-researcher found that melatonin alone (without the other supplements) in a dosage of 6 milligrams taken each night was enough to eliminate symptoms for a woman suffering from severe heartburn.[94]

Finding an "Integrative" Doctor Who May Be More Open to Alternative Approaches

For the name of an integrative doctor, you may wish to consult databases offered by the following organizations listed below. When contacting a physician's office, you could ask whether the doctor does testing for low stomach acid, as very occasionally even an "integrative" physician may not be familiar with this testing or treatment.

- **AMERICAN ASSOCIATION FOR HEALTH FREEDOM**
  www.healthfreedom.net
  1350 Connecticut Ave., NW, 5th Floor
  Washington, D.C. 20036
  For more information:
  office@healthfreedom.net

- **AMERICAN COLLEGE FOR ADVANCEMENT IN MEDICINE**
  www.acam.org
  24411 Ridge Route, Ste 115
  Laguna Hills, CA 92653
  949-309-3520

- **INTERNATIONAL COLLEGE OF INTEGRATIVE MEDICINE**
  www.icimed.com
  122 Thurman Street
  Box 271
  Bluffton, OH 45817
  866-464-5226

- **AMERICAN ACADEMY OF ENVIRONMENTAL MEDICINE**
  www.aaemonline.org
  7701 East Kellogg, Suite 625
  Wichita, KS 67207
  316-684-5500

- **AMERICAN ASSOCIATION OF NATUROPATHIC PHYSICIANS**
  www.naturopathic.org
  4435 Wisconsin Avenue, NW, Suite 403
  Washington, DC 20016
  202-237-8150

- **AMERICAN HOLISTIC MEDICAL ASSOCIATION**
  www.holisticmedicine.org
  One Eagle Valley Court, Suite 201
  Broadview Heights, OH 44147
  440-838-1010

Notes

A Very Widespread Problem

1 Mayo Clinic Website. http://www.mayoclinic .com/health/heartburn-gerd/DS00095 (accessed January 6, 2008). Srinivasan, R., R. Tutuian, P. Schoenfeld, M. F. Vela, J. A. Castell, T. Isaac, I. Galaria, P. O. Katz, and D. O. Castell. 2004. Profile of GERD in the adult population of a northeast urban community. *J Clin Gastroenterol* 38 (8):651–7.

2 Neegaard, L., Complications from Heartburn on the Rise, *Associated Press*, March 31, 2008. Source: American Cancer Society.

3 Kubo, A., T. R. Levin, G. Block, G. J. Rumore, C. P. Quesenberry, Jr., P. Buffler, and D. A. Corley. 2008. Dietary patterns and the risk of Barrett's esophagus. *Am J Epidemiol* 167 (7):839–46.

4 Williams, D. A., Healthy Diet Saves Your Throat, *Alternatives*, March 2008, 69.

We Need Stomach Acid

5 National Institutes of Health. Your Digestive System and How It Works. http://digestive .niddk.nih.gov/ddiseases/pubs/yrdd (accessed January 6, 2008).

6 Wikipedia contributors, Stomach, *Wikipedia, The Free Encyclopedia,* http://en.wikipedia.org/w/ index.php?title=Stomach&oldid=258470505 (accessed January 6, 2008). And a college freshman biology course shows that lowering the acid level in the stomach inhibits digestion of proteins. See http://biology.clc.uc.edu/courses/bio105/ digestiv.html and http://biology.clc.uc.edu/ courses/bio115/pepsin.html (accessed March 27, 2008).

7 Wright, J. and L. Lenard. *Why Stomach Acid Is Good for You: Natural Relief for Heartburn, Indigestion, and GERD* (New York: M. Evans & Company, Inc., 2001), 41.

8 Wright, J. and L. Lenard. *Why Stomach Acid Is Good For You: Natural Relief For Heartburn, Indigestion, and GERD* (New York: M. Evans & Company, Inc., 2001), 79.

Stomach Acid Declines with Age

9 Carey, J., and M. Wetherby. 1941. Gastric observations in achlorhydria. *J Dig Dis* 8:401–407.; also in Geokas, M. C., and B. J. Haverback. 1969. The aging gastrointestinal tract. *Am J Surg* 117 (6):881–92.

Krentz, K., and H. Jablonowski, in *Gastrointestinal Tract Disorders in the Elderly*, ed. J. Hellemans and G. Vantrappen, 62–69 (Edinburgh: Churchill Livingstone, 1984).

Lovat, L. B. 1996. Age related changes in gut physiology and nutritional status. *Gut* 38 (3):306–9.

Russell, R. M. 1992. Changes in gastrointestinal function attributed to aging. *Am J Clin Nutr* 55 (6 Suppl):1203S–1207S.

———. 1997. Gastric hypochlorhydria and achlorhydria in older adults. *JAMA* 278 (20):1659–60.

10 Tanner, L., Digestion Treatments Soar For Kids, *Associated Press*. October 7, 2007, http://www.jsonline.com/story/index.aspx?id=671539 (accessed November 7, 2007).

11 Ibid.

12 Cedars Sinai is a major Los Angeles hospital. Its website discusses this. http://healthinfo.cedars-sinai.edu/library/healthguide/en-us/IllnessConditions/topic.asp? hwid=hw99177 (accessed June 23, 2006). Also cited in *Life Extension, Collectors' Edition 2007*, 85. Also see Wright, J. and L. Lenard. *Why Stomach Acid Is Good For You: Natural Relief for Heartburn, Indigestion, and GERD* (New York: M. Evans & Company, Inc., 2001), 22.

13 Wright, J. and L. Lenard. *Why Stomach Acid Is Good for You: Natural Relief For Heartburn, Indigestion, and GERD* (New York: M. Evans & Company, Inc., 2001), 22.

What Really Causes Heartburn

14 Maher, J. Common Indigestion: Millions of Americans Suffer From It. University of Iowa Health Science Relations. www.uihealthcare.com/topics/medicaldepartments/surgery/gerd/index.html (accessed October 29, 2007).

15 Prilosec OTC Website. What is the cause of heartburn? http://www.prilosecotc.com/heartburn/heartburncauses.jsp (accessed January 14, 2008).

16 GERD Information Resource Center. What is GERD? http://www.gerd.com/consumer/gerd.aspx. (accessed January 14, 2008).

17 American Gastroenterological Association. Heartburn Facts. http://www.gastro.org/wmspage.cfm?parm1=467 (accessed January 11, 2008).

18 Ibid.

What Else Might Cause Acid To Back Up Into the Throat?

19 Higgs, R. H., R. D. Smyth, and D. O. Castell. 1974. Gastric alkalinization. Effect on lower-esophageal-sphincter pressure and serum gastrin. *N Engl J Med* 291 (10):486–90.

20 Castell, D. O., and S. M. Levine. 1971. Lower esophageal sphincter response to gastric alkalinization. A new mechanism for treatment of heartburn with antacids. *Ann Intern Med* 74 (2):223–7.

Freeland, G. R., R. H. Higgs, and D. O. Castell. 1977. Lower esophageal sphincter response to oral administration of cimetidine in normal subjects. *Gastroenterology* 72 (1):28–30.

Kline, M. M., R. W. McCallum, N. Curry, and R. A. Sturdevant. 1975. Effect to gastric alkalinization on lower esophageal sphincter pressure and serum gastrin. *Gastroenterology* 68 (5 Pt 1):1137–9.

McCallum, R. W. 1985. Studies on the mechanism of the lower esophageal sphincter pressure response to alkali ingestion in humans. *Am J Gastroenterol* 80 (7):513–7.

Wallin, L., T. Madsen, M. Brandsborg, O. Brandsborg, and N. E. Larsen. 1979. The influence of cimetidine on basal gastro-oesophageal sphincter pressure, intargastric pH, and serum gastrin concentration in normal subjects. *Scand J Gastroenterol* 14 (3):349–53.

21 Health Sciences Institute. Preventing Esophageal Cancer. http://www.hsibaltimore.com/ealerts/ea200503/ea20050315.html (accessed January 11, 2008).

Spreen, A., Healthnews.com. November 4, 2004, 1–2 and November 11, 2004, 1–2; also cited in Dr. James Howenstine, The Health Risks of Blocking Acid Production by the Stomach. December 9, 2004. http://www.newswithviews.com/howenstine/james21html (accessed June 3, 2007).

Why Antacids Might Make the Situation Worse

22 For a very detailed summary of many scientific studies that support this idea, see Steinnon, O. Arthur MD, Reflex control of the sphincter, in *The Longitudinal Muscle in Esophageal Disease*. (Radiology Publishing, 1995), http://www.esophagushoncho.com (accessed March 17, 2008).

23 Mayo Clinic Website. http://www.mayoclinic
.com/health/heartburn-gerd/DS00095 (Accessed
July 8, 2006). *Cited by Life Extension, Collector's
Edition, 2007, 84.*

What Is Really Happening?

24 Lyman, H. M. 1897. Chronic catarrhal gastritis. *JAMA* 28(8):439–442.

25 Azpiroz, F. Understanding Intestinal Gas. International Foundation for Functional Gastrointestinal Disorders. https://www.iffgd.org/store/
downloadfile/214 (accessed January 4, 2008.

Doesn't Everybody "Know" that Antacids Are the Stomach Medicine of Choice?

26 IMS Health. IMS World Review 2004, summary
information provided at http://www.imshealth
.com/web/content/0,1348, 64576068_63872702
_70260998_70960214,00.html (accessed January
15, 2008.

27 Visiongain. Gastrointestinal Disorders Market
Intelligence to 2012. May 25, 2007.

28 AstraZeneca Annual Report 2006. http://
www.astrazeneca.com/sites/7/imagebank/
typeArticleparam511715/astrazeneca-annual-
report-20F-2006.pdf (accessed January 10, 2008).

29 Center for Public Integrity. Drug Lobby Second to
None: How the Pharmaceutical Industry Gets Its
Way in Washington. http://www.publicintegrity
.org/rx/report.aspx?aid=723 (accessed March 20,
2008).

What Drug Companies Actually Say

30 Wright, J. and L. Lenard. *Why Stomach Acid Is Good for You: Natural Relief For Heartburn, Indigestion, and GERD* (New York: M. Evans & Company, Inc., 2001), 23.

31 Prilosec OTC Website. What does heartburn feel like? www.prilosecotc.com/heartburn/symptoms.jsp (accessed March 19, 2008).

32 AstraZeneca Website. Prilosec Prescribing Information. http://www.astrazeneca-us.com/pi/Prilosec.pdf (accessed January 14, 2008).

33 National Heartburn Alliance. Get Heartburn Smart. http://www.heartburnalliance.org/pdfs/brochure.pdf (accessed December 10, 2007).

34 Mayo Clinic Health Letter. 2006. If stomach acid helps digest food, how is food digested if you take an antacid after a meal? *Mayo Clin Health Lett* March 24(3):8.

35 Maton, P. N. 2003. Profile and assessment of GERD pharmacotherapy. *Cleve Clin J Med* 70 Suppl 5:S51–70.

36 AstraZeneca Website. Prescribing Information. http://www.astrazeneca-us.com/pi/Nexium.pdf and http://www.astrazeneca-us.com/pi/Prilosec.pdf (accessed January 14, 2008).

Don't Many Doctors Agree with the Drug Companies?

37 Angell, M. 2000. Is academic medicine for sale? *N Engl J Med* 342 (20):1516–8.

Boyd, E. A., and L. A. Bero. 2000. Assessing faculty financial relationships with industry: A case study. *JAMA* 284 (17):2209–14.

Cho, M. K., R. Shohara, A. Schissel, and D. Rennie. 2000. Policies on faculty conflicts of interest at US universities. *JAMA* 284 (17):2203–8.

Doesn't the Government Support the Use of Antacids?

38 Angell, M. 2000. The pharmaceutical industry—to whom is it accountable? *N Engl J Med* 342 (25):1902–4.

Center for Science in the Public Interest. Conflicts of Interest on Cox-2 Panel. http://www.cspinet.org/new/200502251html (accessed January 28, 2008).

39 Food and Drug Administration Amendments Act of 2007. http://www.fda.gov/oc/initiatives/HR3580.pdf (accessed January 28, 2008).

40 Schmit, J., Bush Budget Plan's Drug Fees Attacked, *USA Today*, February 14, 2007. http://www.usatoday.com/money/industries/health/drugs/2007-02-14-fda-budget-usat_x.html (accessed January 28, 2008).

Rubin, R., FDA Called 'Cozy' with Drugmakers, *USA Today*. http://www.usatoday.com/news/health/2007-06-11-fda-drugmakers_N.htm?csp=34&POE=click-refer (accessed March 20, 2008).

Why Antacids May Be Bad for Your Bones

41 Allison, J. R. 1945. The relation of hydrochloric acid and vitamin B complex deficiency in certain skin diseases. *South Med J* 38:235.

Kassarjian, Z., and R. M. Russell. 1989. Hypochlorhydria: a factor in nutrition. *Annu Rev Nutr* 9:271–85.

Maltby, E. J. 1934. The Digestion of Beef Proteins in the Human Stomach. *J Clin Invest* 13 (2):193–207.

Ogilvie, J. 1935. The gastric secretion in anaemia. *Arch Dis Childhood* 10:143–148.

42 Yang, Y. X., J. D. Lewis, S. Epstein, and D. C. Metz. 2006. Long-term proton pump inhibitor therapy and risk of hip fracture. *JAMA* 296 (24):2947–53.

43 Insogna, K. L., D. R. Bordley, J. F. Caro, and D. H. Lockwood. 1980. Osteomalacia and weakness from excessive antacid ingestion. *JAMA* 244 (22):2544–6.

Saadeh, G., T. Bauer, A. Licata, and L. Sheeler. 1987. Antacid-induced osteomalacia. *Cleve Clin J Med* 54 (3):214–6.

44 Robertson, D. S. 2005. The chemical reactions in the human stomach and the relationship to metabolic disorders. *Med Hypotheses* 64 (6):1127–31.

Robinson, R. F., M. J. Casavant, M. C. Nahata, and J. D. Mahan. 2004. Metabolic bone disease after chronic antacid administration in an infant. *Ann Pharmacother* 38 (2):265–8.

Spencer, H., and L. Kramer. 1985. Osteoporosis: calcium, fluoride, and aluminum interactions. *J Am Coll Nutr* 4 (1):121–8.

45 Bo-Linn, G. W., G. R. Davis, D. J. Buddrus, S. G. Morawski, C. Santa Ana, and J. S. Fordtran. 1984. An evaluation of the importance of gastric acid secretion in the absorption of dietary calcium. *J Clin Invest* 73 (3):640–7.

Ivanovich, P., H. Fellows, and C. Rich. 1967. The absorption of calcium carbonate. *Ann Intern Med* 66 (5):917–23.

O'Connell, M. B., D. M. Madden, A. M. Murray, R. P. Heaney, and L. J. Kerzner. 2005. Effects of proton pump inhibitors on calcium carbonate absorption in women: a randomized crossover trial. *Am J Med* 118 (7):778–81.

Recker, R. R. 1985. Calcium absorption and achlorhydria. *N Engl J Med* 313 (2):70–3.

Spencer, H., L. Kramer, C. Norris, and D. Osis. 1982. Effect of small doses of aluminum-containing antacids on calcium and phosphorus metabolism. *Am J Clin Nutr* 36 (1):32–40.

Wood, R., and C. Serfaty-Lacrosniere. Effects of gastric acidity and atrophic gastritis on calcium and zinc absorption in humans, in *Chronic Gastritis and Hypochlorhydria in the Elderly*, ed. P. Holt and R. Russell, 187–204 (Boca Raton, FL: CRC Press, 1993).

Other Medical Conditions Associated with Low Stomach Acid

46 Bezwoda, W., R. Charlton, T. Bothwell, J. Torrance, and F. Mayet. 1978. The importance of gastric hydrochloric acid in the absorption of non-heme food iron. *J Lab Clin Med* 92 (1):108–16.

Jacobs, A., J. H. Lawrie, C. C. Entwistle, and H. Campbell. 1966. Gastric acid secretion in chronic iron-deficiency anaemia. *Lancet* 2 (7456):190–2.

Jacobs, P., T. Bothwell, and R. W. Charlton. 1964. Role of Hydrochloric Acid in Iron Absorption. *J Appl Physiol* 19:187–8.

Lazlo, J., Effect of gastrointestinal conditions on the mineral-binding properties of dietary fibers: in *Mineral Absorption in the Monogastric GI Tract (Advances in Experimental Medicine and Biology, Vol 249)*, ed. F. Dintzis and J. Lazlo (New York: Plenum Press, 1993).

Marcuard, S. P., L. Albernaz, and P. G. Khazanie. 1994. Omeprazole therapy causes malabsorption of cyanocobalamin (vitamin B12). *Ann Intern Med* 120 (3):211–5.

McCarthy, C. F. 1976. Nutritional defects in patients with malabsorption. *Proc Nutr Soc* 35 (1):37–40.

Murray, M. J., and N. Stein. 1968. A gastric factor promoting iron absorption. *Lancet* 1 (7543):614–6.

O'Neil-Cutting, M. A., and W. H. Crosby. 1986. The effect of antacids on the absorption of simultaneously ingested iron. *JAMA* 255 (11):1468–70.

Pedrosa, M., and R. Russell, Folate and vitamin B12 absorption in atrophic gastritis, in *Chronic*

Gastritis and Hypochlorhydria in the Elderly, ed. P. Holt and R. Russell, 157–169 (Boca Raton, FL: CRC Press, 1993).

Russell, R. M., B. B. Golner, S. D. Krasinski, J. A. Sadowski, P. M. Suter, and C. L. Braun. 1988. Effect of antacid and H2 receptor antagonists on the intestinal absorption of folic acid. *J Lab Clin Med* 112 (4):458–63.

Saltzman, J. R., J. A. Kemp, B. B. Golner, M. C. Pedrosa, G. E. Dallal, and R. M. Russell. 1994. Effect of hypochlorhydria due to omeprazole treatment or atrophic gastritis on protein-bound vitamin B12 absorption. *J Am Coll Nutr* 13 (6):584–91.

Shindo, K., M. Machida, M. Fukumura, K. Koide, and R. Yamazaki. 1998. Omeprazole induces altered bile acid metabolism. *Gut* 42 (2):266–71.

Skikne, B. S., S. R. Lynch, and J. D. Cook. 198 1 Role of gastric acid in food iron absorption. *Gastroenterology* 81 (6):1068–71.

Steinberg, W. M., C. E. King, and P. P. Toskes. 1980. Malabsorption of protein-bound cobalamin but not unbound cobalamin during cimetidine administration. *Dig Dis Sci* 25 (3):188–91.

Sturniolo, G. C., M. C. Montino, L. Rossetto, A. Martin, R. D'Inca, A. D'Odorico, and R. Naccarato. 199 1 Inhibition of gastric acid secretion reduces zinc absorption in man. *J Am Coll Nutr* 10 (4):372–5.

Vagnini, F., and B. Fox, Preventing pharmaceutical-induced nutritional deficiencies *Life Extension* March 2006, 72–9.

47 Dial, S., J. A. Delaney, A. N. Barkun, and S. Suissa. 2005. Use of gastric acid-suppressive agents and the risk of community-acquired Clostridium difficile-associated disease. *JAMA* 294 (23):2989–95.

Dial, S., J. A. Delaney, V. Schneider, and S. Suissa. 2006. Proton pump inhibitor use and risk of community-acquired Clostridium difficile-associated disease defined by prescription for oral vancomycin therapy. *CMAJ* 175 (7):745–8.

48 Clemons, T. E., R. C. Milton, R. Klein, J. M. Seddon, and F. L. Ferris, 3rd. 2005. Risk factors for the incidence of Advanced Age-Related Macular Degeneration in the Age-Related Eye Disease Study (AREDS) AREDS report no. 19. *Ophthalmology* 112 (4):533–9.

Douglas, I. J., C. Cook, U. Chakravarthy, R. Hubbard, A. E. Fletcher, and L. Smeeth. 2007. A case-control study of drug risk factors for age-related macular degeneration. *Ophthalmology* 114 (6):1164–9.

49 Boustani, M., K. S. Hall, K. A. Lane, H. Aljadhey, S. Gao, F. Unverzagt, M. D. Murray, A. Ogunniyi, and H. Hendrie. 2007. The association between cognition and histamine-2 receptor antagonists in African Americans. *J Am Geriatr Soc* 55 (8):1248–53.

50 Kodama, K., K. Sumii, M. Kawano, T. Kido, K. Nojima, M. Sumii, K. Haruma, M. Yoshihara, and K. Chayama. 2003. Gastric juice nitrite and vitamin C in patients with gastric cancer and atrophic gastritis: is low acidity solely responsible

for cancer risk? *Eur J Gastroenterol Hepatol* 15 (9):987–93.

Sobala, G. M., C. J. Schorah, B. Pignatelli, J. E. Crabtree, I. G. Martin, N. Scott, and P. Quirke. 1993. High gastric juice ascorbic acid concentrations in members of a gastric cancer family. *Carcinogenesis* 14 (2):291–2.

Sobala, G. M., C. J. Schorah, M. Sanderson, M. F. Dixon, D. S. Tompkins, P. Godwin, and A. T. Axon. 1989. Ascorbic acid in the human stomach. *Gastroenterology* 97 (2):357–63.

51 Canani, R. B., P. Cirillo, P. Roggero, C. Romano, B. Malamisura, G. Terrin, A. Passariello, F. Manguso, L. Morelli, and A. Guarino. 2006. Therapy with gastric acidity inhibitors increases the risk of acute gastroenteritis and community-acquired pneumonia in children. *Pediatrics* 117 (5):e817–20.

———. 2006. Therapy with gastric acidity inhibitors increases the risk of acute gastroenteritis and community-acquired pneumonia in children. *Pediatrics* 117 (5):e817–20.

Driks, M. R., D. E. Craven, B. R. Celli, M. Manning, R. A. Burke, G. M. Garvin, L. M. Kunches, H. W. Farber, S. A. Wedel, and W. R. McCabe. 1987. Nosocomial pneumonia in intubated patients given sucralfate as compared with antacids or histamine type 2 blockers. The role of gastric colonization. *N Engl J Med* 317 (22):1376–82.

Federico, M. 2005. Does treating gastroesophageal reflux cause pneumonia? *J Pediatr Gastroenterol Nutr* 40 (3):386–7.

Gregor, J. C. 2004. Acid suppression and pneumonia: a clinical indication for rational prescribing. *JAMA* 292 (16):2012–3.

Laheij, R. J., M. C. Sturkenboom, R. J. Hassing, J. Dieleman, B. H. Stricker, and J. B. Jansen. 2004. Risk of community-acquired pneumonia and use of gastric acid-suppressive drugs. *JAMA* 292 (16):1955–60.

Laheij, R. J., M. C. Van Ijzendoorn, M. J. Janssen, and J. B. Jansen. 2003. Gastric acid-suppressive therapy and community-acquired respiratory infections. *Aliment Pharmacol Ther* 18 (8):847–51.

Nitschmann, S. 2006. [Increased risk of pneumonia through gastric acid reduction. Partial evaluation of the Integrated Primary Care Information Project (IPCIP)]. *Internist (Berl)* 47 (4):441–2; discussion 442.

Sataloff, R. T. 2005. Community-acquired pneumonia and use of gastric acid-suppressive drugs. *JAMA* 293 (7):795–6; author reply 796.

52 Colorado State University Website. Pathophysiology of the Digestive System. http://arbl.cvmbs.colostate.edu/hbooks/pathphys/digestion (accessed February 29, 2008).

53 Fried, M., H. Siegrist, R. Frei, F. Froehlich, P. Duroux, J. Thorens, A. Blum, J. Bille, J. J. Gonvers, and K. Gyr. 1994. Duodenal bacterial overgrowth during treatment in outpatients with omeprazole. *Gut* 35 (1):23–6.

Garcia Rodriguez, L. A., and A. Ruigomez. 1997. Gastric acid, acid-suppressing drugs, and bacterial gastroenteritis: how much of a risk? *Epidemiology* 8 (5):571–4.

Gitelson, S. 1971. Gastrectomy, achlorhydria and cholera. *Isr J Med Sci* 7 (5):663–7.

Goddard, A. F., and R. C. Spiller. 1996. The effect of omeprazole on gastric juice viscosity, pH and bacterial counts. *Aliment Pharmacol Ther* 10 (1):105–9.

Goldin, B., and S. Gorbach, Bacterial overgrowth in atrophic gastritis, in *Chronic Gastritis and Hypochlorhydria in the Elderly*, ed. P. Holt and R. Russell, 143–156 (Boca Raton, FL: CRC Press, 1993).

Gough, A., D. Andrews, P. A. Bacon, and P. Emery. 1995. Evidence of omeprazole-induced small bowel bacterial overgrowth in patients with scleroderma. *Br J Rheumatol* 34 (10):976–7.

Lewis, S. J., S. Franco, G. Young, and S. J. O'Keefe. 1996. Altered bowel function and duodenal bacterial overgrowth in patients treated with omeprazole. *Aliment Pharmacol Ther* 10 (4):557–61.

Patel, T. A., P. Abraham, V. J. Ashar, S. J. Bhatia, and P. S. Anklesaria. 1995. Gastric bacterial overgrowth accompanies profound acid suppression. *Indian J Gastroenterol* 14 (4):134–6.

Pereira, S. P., N. Gainsborough, and R. H. Dowling. 1998. Drug-induced hypochlorhydria causes high duodenal bacterial counts in the elderly. *Aliment Pharmacol Ther* 12 (1):99–104.

Peura, D., and R. Guerrant, Achlorhydria and enteric bacteria infections, in *Chronic Gastritis and Hypochlorhydria in the Elderly*, ed. P. Holt and R. Russell, 127–142 (Boca Raton, FL: CRC Press, 1993).

Saltzman, J. R., K. V. Kowdley, M. C. Pedrosa, T. Sepe, B. Golner, G. Perrone, and R. M. Russell. 1994. Bacterial overgrowth without clinical malabsorption in elderly hypochlorhydric subjects. *Gastroenterology* 106 (3):615–23.

Van Loon, F. P., J. D. Clemens, M. Shahrier, D. A. Sack, C. B. Stephensen, M. R. Khan, G. H. Rabbani, M. R. Rao, and A. K. Banik. 1990. Low gastric acid as a risk factor for cholera transmission: application of a new non-invasive gastric acid field test. *J Clin Epidemiol* 43 (12):1361–7.

54 Karmeli, Y., R. Stalnikowitz, R. Eliakim, and G. Rahav. 1995. Conventional dose of omeprazole alters gastric flora. *Dig Dis Sci* 40 (9):2070–3.

55 Sarela, A. I., D. G. Hick, C. S. Verbeke, J. F. Casey, P. J. Guillou, and G. W. Clark. "Persistent Acid and Bile Reflux in Asymptomatic Patients with Barrett Esophagus Receiving Proton Pump Inhibitor Therapy." *Arch Surg* 139, no. 5 (2004): 547-51.

Theisen, J., D. Nehra, D. Citron, J. Johansson, J. A. Hagen, P. F. Crookes, S. R. DeMeester, C. G. Bremner, T. R. DeMeester, and J. H. Peters. "Suppression of Gastric Acid Secretion in Patients with Gastroesophageal Reflux Disease Results in Gastric Bacterial Overgrowth and Deconjugation of Bile Acids." *J Gastrointest Surg* 4, no. 1 (2000): 50-4.

See also Mayo Clinic Website http://www.mayoclinic.com (accessed January 6, 2008) re link between bile reflux and esophageal cancer.

56 Nalin, D. R., R. J. Levine, M. M. Levine, D. Hoover, E. Bergquist, J. McLaughlin, J. Libonati,

J. Alam, and R. B. Hornick. 1978. Cholera, non-vibrio cholera, and stomach acid. *Lancet* 2 (8095):856–9.

Antacids and Stomach Ulcers

57 Australian Institute of Policy and Science. Barry Marshall: Gastroenterologist. http://www .tallpoppies.net.au/cavalcade/marshall.html (accessed September 9, 2006).

Blaser, M. J. 1996. The bacteria behind ulcers. *Sci Am* 274 (2):104–7.

Kuipers, E. J., J. C. Thijs, and H. P. Festen. 1995. The prevalence of *Helicobacter pylori* in peptic ulcer disease. *Aliment Pharmacol Ther* 9 Suppl 2:59–69.

Marshall, B. J. Unidentified curved bacillus on gastric epithelium in active chronic gastritis. *Lancet* 1 (8336):1273–1275.

Marshall, B. J, and J. R. Warren. Unidentified curved bacilli in the stomach patients with gastritis and peptic ulceration. *Lancet* 1 (8390):1311–1315.

Riccardi, V. M., and J. I. Rotter. 1994. Familial *Helicobacter pylori* infection. Societal factors, human genetics, and bacterial genetics. *Ann Intern Med* 120 (12):1043–5.

58 An international association between *Helicobacter pylori* infection and gastric cancer. The EUROGAST Study Group. 1993. *Lancet* 341 (8857):1359–62.

Bayerdorffer, E., A. Neubauer, B. Rudolph, C. Thiede, N. Lehn, S. Eidt, and M. Stolte. 1995.

Regression of primary gastric lymphoma of mucosa-associated lymphoid tissue type after cure of *Helicobacter pylori* infection. MALT Lymphoma Study Group. *Lancet* 345 (8965):1591–4.

De Koster, E., M. Buset, E. Fernandes, and M. Deltenre. 1994. *Helicobacter pylori*: the link with gastric cancer. *Eur J Cancer Prev* 3 (3):247–57.

Fendrick, A. M., M. E. Chernew, R. A. Hirth, B. S. Bloom, R. R. Bandekar, and J. M. Scheiman. 1999. Clinical and economic effects of population-based *Helicobacter pylori* screening to prevent gastric cancer. *Arch Intern Med* 159 (2):142–8.

Forman, D., D. G. Newell, F. Fullerton, J. W. Yarnell, A. R. Stacey, N. Wald, and F. Sitas. 1991. Association between infection with *Helicobacter pylori* and risk of gastric cancer: evidence from a prospective investigation. *BMJ* 302 (6788):1302–5.

Hansson, L. E., O. Nyren, A. W. Hsing, R. Bergstrom, S. Josefsson, W. H. Chow, J. F. Fraumeni, Jr., and H. O. Adami. 1996. The risk of stomach cancer in patients with gastric or duodenal ulcer disease. *N Engl J Med* 335 (4):242–9.

Henschel E., G. Brandstatter, B. Dragosics et al. 1993. Effect of ranitidine and amoxicillin plus metronidazole on the eradication of Helcobacter pylori and the recurrence of duodenal ulcer. *New Engl J Med* 328:308–312.

Kuipers, E. J., A. S. Pena, and S. G. Meuwissen. 1995. [*Helicobacter pylori* infection as causal factor in the development of carcinoma and lymphoma of the stomach; report WHO consensus conference]. *Ned Tijdschr Geneeskd* 139 (14):709–12.

Kuipers, E. J., A. M. Uyterlinde, A. S. Pena, R. Roosendaal, G. Pals, G. F. Nelis, H. P. Festen, and S. G. Meuwissen. 1995. Long-term sequelae of *Helicobacter pylori* gastritis. *Lancet* 345 (8964):1525–8.

Mertz, H., *Helicobacter pylori*: Its role in gastritis, achlorhydria, and gastric carcinoma in *Chronic Gastritis and Hypochlorhydria in the Elderly*, ed. P. Holt and R. Russell, 69–82 (Boca Raton, FL: CRC Press, 1993).

Munoz, N. 1994. Is *Helicobacter pylori* a cause of gastric cancer? An appraisal of the seroepidemiological evidence. *Cancer Epidemiol Biomarkers Prev* 3 (5):445–51.

Murakami, K., M. Kodama, and T. Fujioka. 2006. Latest insights into the effects of *Helicobacter pylori* infection on gastric carcinogenesis. *World J Gastroenterol* 12 (17):2713–20.

Nomura, A., G. N. Stemmermann, P. H. Chyou, I. Kato, G. I. Perez-Perez, and M. J. Blaser. 1991. *Helicobacter pylori* infection and gastric carcinoma among Japanese Americans in Hawaii. *N Engl J Med* 325 (16):1132–6.

Parsonnet, J., G. D. Friedman, D. P. Vandersteen, Y. Chang, J. H. Vogelman, N. Orentreich, and R. K. Sibley. 1991. *Helicobacter pylori* infection and the risk of gastric carcinoma. *N Engl J Med* 325 (16):1127–31.

Suzuki, T., K. Matsuo, H. Ito, K. Hirose, K. Wakai, T. Saito, S. Sato, Y. Morishima, S. Nakamura,

R. Ueda, and K. Tajima. 2006. A past history of gastric ulcers and *Helicobacter pylori* infection increase the risk of gastric malignant lymphoma. *Carcinogenesis* 27 (7):1391–7.

Uemura, N., T. Mukai, S. Okamoto, S. Yamaguchi, H. Mashiba, K. Taniyama, N. Sasaki, K. Haruma, K. Sumii, and G. Kajiyama. 1997. Effect of *Helicobacter pylori* eradication on subsequent development of cancer after endoscopic resection of early gastric cancer. *Cancer Epidemiol Biomarkers Prev* 6 (8):639–42.

Wotherspoon, A. C., C. Doglioni, T. C. Diss, L. Pan, A. Moschini, M. de Boni, and P. G. Isaacson. 1993. Regression of primary low-grade B-cell gastric lymphoma of mucosa-associated lymphoid tissue type after eradication of *Helicobacter pylori*. *Lancet* 342 (8871):575–7.

Zucca, E., F. Bertoni, E. Roggero, G. Bosshard, G. Cazzaniga, E. Pedrinis, A. Biondi, and F. Cavalli. 1998. Molecular analysis of the progression from *Helicobacter pylori*-associated chronic gastritis to mucosa-associated lymphoid-tissue lymphoma of the stomach. *N Engl J Med* 338 (12):804–10.

59 Argent, R. H., R. J. Thomas, F. Aviles-Jimenez, D. P. Letley, M. C. Limb, E. M. El-Omar, and J. C. Atherton. 2008. Toxigenic *Helicobacter pylori* infection precedes gastric hypochlorhydria in cancer relatives, and *H. pylori* virulence evolves in these families. *Clin Cancer Res* 14 (7):2227–35.

Borody T., T. Noonan, P. Cole et al. 1989. Triple therapy of C. pylori can reverse hypochlorhydria. *Am J Gastroenterology* 96:A53.

Cater, R. E., 2nd. 1992. The clinical importance of hypochlorhydria (a consequence of chronic Helicobacter infection): its possible etiological role in mineral and amino acid malabsorption, depression, and other syndromes. *Med Hypotheses* 39 (4):375–83.

———. 1992. Helicobacter (aka Campylobacter) pylori as the major causal factor in chronic hypochlorhydria. *Med Hypotheses* 39 (4):367–74.

Iijima, K., H. Sekine, T. Koike, A. Imatani, S. Ohara, and T. Shimosegawa. 2004. Long-term effect of *Helicobacter pylori* eradication on the reversibility of acid secretion in profound hypochlorhydria. *Aliment Pharmacol Ther* 19 (11):1181–8.

Schubert, M. L. 2002. Gastric secretion. *Curr Opin Gastroenterol* 18 (6):639–49.

Xia, H. H., and N. J. Talley. 1998. *Helicobacter pylori* infection, reflux esophagitis, and atrophic gastritis: an unexplored triangle. *Am J Gastroenterol* 93 (3):394–400.

60 Bloomfield, A., and W. Polland, Anacidity with cancer of the stomach, in *Gastric Anacidity: Its Relation to Disease*, 125–136 (New York: MacMillan, 1933).

Christiansen, P. M. 1968. The incidence of achlorhydria and hypochlorhydria in healthy subjects and patients with gastrointestinal diseases. *Scand J Gastroenterol* 3 (5):497–508.

Kuster, G. G., W. H. ReMine, and M. B. Dockerty. 1972. Gastric cancer in pernicious anemia and in patients with and without achlorhydria. *Ann Surg* 175 (5):783–9.

Morgan, J. E., C. W. Kaiser, W. Johnson, W. G. Doos, Y. Dayal, L. Berman, and D. Nabseth. 1983. Gastric carcinoid (gastrinoma) associated with achlorhydria (pernicious anemia). *Cancer* 51 (12):2332–40.

Segal, H. L., and I. M. Samloff. 1973. Gastric cancer—increased frequency in patients with achlorhydria. *Am J Dig Dis* 18 (4):295–9.

61 Al-Habbal, M. J., Z. Al-Habbal, and F. U. Huwez. 1984. A double-blind controlled clinical trial of mastic and placebo in the treatment of duodenal ulcer. *Clin Exp Pharmacol Physiol* 11 (5):541–4.

Al-Said, M. S., A. M. Ageel, N. S. Parmar, and M. Tariq. 1986. Evaluation of mastic, a crude drug obtained from Pistacia lentiscus for gastric and duodenal anti-ulcer activity. *J Ethnopharmacol* 15 (3):271–8.

Huwez, F. U., D. Thirlwell, A. Cockayne, and D. A. Ala'Aldeen. 1998. Mastic gum kills *Helicobacter pylori*. *N Engl J Med* 339 (26):1946.

62 Cheney, G. 1949. Rapid healing of peptic ulcers in patients receiving fresh cabbage juice. *Calif Med* 70 (1):10–5.

———. 1952. Vitamin U therapy of peptic ulcer. *Calif Med* 77 (4):248–52.

Cheney, G., S. H. Waxler, and I. J. Miller. 1956. Vitamin U therapy of peptic ulcer; experience at San Quentin Prison. *Calif Med* 84 (1):39–42.

Doll, R., and F. Pygott. 1954. Clinical trial of Robaden and of cabbage juice in the treatment of gastric ulcer. *Lancet* 267 (6850):1200–4.

Vargha, G., and F. Damrau. 1963. Standardized cabbage factor complex for peptic ulcers. Report of animal experiments and 162 ambulatory cases. *J Am Med Womens Assoc* 18:460–3.

63 Jones, N. L., S. Shabib, and P. M. Sherman. 1997. Capsaicin as an inhibitor of the growth of the gastric pathogen *Helicobacter pylori*. *FEMS Microbiol Lett* 146 (2):223–7.

Satyanarayana, M. N. 2006. Capsaicin and gastric ulcers. *Crit Rev Food Sci Nutr* 46 (4):275–328.

64 Bardhan, K. D., D. C. Cumberland, R. A. Dixon, and C. D. Holdsworth. 1978. Clinical trial of deglycyrrhizinised liquorice in gastric ulcer. *Gut* 19 (9):779–82.

Doll, R., and I. D. Hill. 1962. Triterpenoid liquorice compound in gastric and duodenal ulcer. *Lancet* 2 (7266):1166–7.

Engqvist, A., F. von Feilitzen, E. Pyk, and H. Reichard. 1973. Double-blind trial of deglycyrrhizinated liquorice in gastric ulcer. *Gut* 14 (9):711–5.

Feldman, H., and T. Gilat. 1971. A trial of deglycyrrhizinated liquorice in the treatment of duodenal ulcer. *Gut* 12 (6):449–51.

Fuhrman, B., S. Buch, J. Vaya, P. A. Belinky, R. Coleman, T. Hayek, and M. Aviram. 1997. Licorice extract and its major polyphenol glabridin protect low-density lipoprotein against lipid peroxidation: in vitro and ex vivo studies in humans and in atherosclerotic apolipoprotein E-deficient mice. *Am J Clin Nutr* 66 (2):267–75.

Fukai, T., A. Marumo, K. Kaitou, T. Kanda, S. Terada, and T. Nomura. 2002. Anti-*Helicobacter pylori* flavonoids from licorice extract. *Life Sci* 71 (12):1449–63.

Glick, L. 1982. Deglycyrrhizinated liquorice for peptic ulcer. *Lancet* 2 (8302):817.

Hollanders, D., G. Green, I. L. Woolf, B. E. Boyes, R. Y. Wilson, D. J. Cowley, and I. W. Dymock. 1978. Prophylaxis with deglycyrrhizinised liquorice in patients with healed gastric ulcer. *Br Med J* 1 (6106):148.

Kassir, Z. A. 1985. Endoscopic controlled trial of four drug regimens in the treatment of chronic duodenal ulceration. *Ir Med J* 78 (6):153–6.

Larkworthy, W., P. F. Holgate, M. B. McIllmurray, and M. J. Langman. 1977. Deglycyrrhizinised liquorice in duodenal ulcer. *Br Med J* 2 (6095):1123.

Morgan, R. J. et al. 1982. The effect of deglycyrrhizinized liquorice on the occurrence of aspirin and aspirin plus bile acid-induced gastric lesions, and aspirin absorption in rats. *Gastroenterology* 82:1134.

Pompei, R., O. Flore, M. A. Marccialis, A. Pani, and B. Loddo. 1979. Glycyrrhizic acid inhibits virus growth and inactivates virus particles. *Nature* 281 (5733):689–90.

Rees, W. D., J. Rhodes, J. E. Wright, L. F. Stamford, and A. Bennett. 1979. Effect of deglycyrrhizinated liquorice on gastric mucosal damage by aspirin. *Scand J Gastroenterol* 14 (5):605–7.

Russell, R. I., and J. E. N. Dickie. 1968. Clinical trial of a deglycyrrhizinized liquorice preparation in peptic ulcer. *J Ther Clin Res* 2:2.

Russell, R. I., R. J. Morgan, and L. M. Nelson. 1984. Studies on the protective effect of deglycyrrhinised liquorice against aspirin (ASA) and ASA plus bile acid-induced gastric mucosal damage, and ASA absorption in rats. *Scand J Gastroenterol Suppl* 92:97–100.

Tewari, S. N., and A. K. Wilson. 1972. Deglycyrrhizinated liquorice in duodenal ulcer. *Practitioner* 210:820.

Turpie, A. G., J. Runcie, and T. J. Thomson. 1969. Clinical trial of deglydyrrhizinized liquorice in gastric ulcer. *Gut* 10 (4):299–302.

van Marle, J. et al. 1981 Deglycyrrhizinised liquorice (DGL) and the renewal of rat stomach epithelium. *Eur J Pharmcol* 72:219–225.

Yoshikawa, M., Y. Matsui, H. Kawamoto, N. Umemoto, K. Oku, M. Koizumi, J. Yamao, S. Kuriyama, H. Nakano, N. Hozumi, S. Ishizaka, and H. Fukui. 1997. Effects of glycyrrhizin on immune-mediated cytotoxicity. *J Gastroenterol Hepatol* 12 (3):243–8.

65 Khuylusi, S. 1995. The effect of unsaturated fatty acids on *Helicobacter pylori* in vitro. *M Med Micro* 42(4):276–282.

Romero, C., E. Medina, J. Vargas, M. Brenes, and A. De Castro. 2007. In vitro activity of olive oil polyphenols against *Helicobacter pylori*. *J Agric Food Chem* 55 (3):680–6.

66 Bone, K. Eleven things you can eat or drink to knock out the hidden factor behind chronic—even deadly—disease. *Nutrition & Healing*, March 2005, 8.

Arora, A., and M. P. Sharma. 1990. Use of banana in non-ulcer dyspepsia. *Lancet* 335 (8689):612–3.

Sikka, K. K. et al. 1988. Efficacy of dried raw banana powder in the healing of peptic ulcer. *J Assoc Physicians India* 36:65–66.

Bullock, C. 1984. Can plantains prevent ulcers? *Med Tribune* 25(33):3.

Rafatullah, S., M. Tariq, M. A. Al-Yahya, J. S. Mossa, and A. M. Ageel. 1990. Evaluation of turmeric (Curcuma longa) for gastric and duodenal antiulcer activity in rats. *J Ethnopharmacol* 29 (1):25–34.

Kositchaiwat, C., S. Kositchaiwat, and J. Havanondha. 1993. Curcuma longa Linn. in the treatment of gastric ulcer comparison to liquid antacid: a controlled clinical trial. *J Med Assoc Thai* 76 (11):601–5.

Glavin, G. B. 1933. Ascorbic acid and cold restraint ulcer in rats: dose-response relationship. *Nutr Rep Int* 28:705.

Jarosz, M., J. Dzieniszewski, E. Dabrowska-Ufniarz, M. Wartanowicz, S. Ziemlanski, and P. I. Reed. 1998. Effects of high dose vitamin C treatment on *Helicobacter pylori* infection and total vitamin C concentration in gastric juice. *Eur J Cancer Prev* 7 (6):449–54.

Zhang, H. M., N. Wakisaka, O. Maeda, and T. Yamamoto. 1997. Vitamin C inhibits the growth of a bacterial risk factor for gastric carcinoma: *Helicobacter pylori*. *Cancer* 80 (10):1897–903.

Zullo, A., V. Rinaldi, C. Hassan, F. Diana, S. Winn, G. Castagna, and A. F. Attili. 2000. Ascorbic acid and intestinal metaplasia in the stomach: a prospective, randomized study. *Aliment Pharmacol Ther* 14 (10):1303–9.

Bandyopadhyay, D., K. Biswas, M. Bhattacharyya, R. J. Reiter, and R. K. Banerjee. 2001. Gastric toxicity and mucosal ulceration induced by oxygen-derived reactive species: protection by melatonin. *Curr Mol Med* 1 (4):501–13.

Bandyopadhyay, D., A. Bandyopadhyay, P. K. Das, and R. J. Reiter. 2002. Melatonin protects against gastric ulceration and increases the efficacy of ranitidine and omeprazole in reducing gastric damage. *J Pineal Res* 33 (1):1–7.

Bandyopadhyay, D., G. Ghosh, A. Bandyopadhyay, and R. J. Reiter. 2004. Melatonin protects against piroxicam-induced gastric ulceration. *J Pineal Res* 36 (3):195–203.

Bandyopadhyay, D., and A. Chattopadhyay. 2006. Reactive oxygen species-induced gastric ulceration: protection by melatonin. *Curr Med Chem* 13 (10):1187–202.

de Souza Pereira, R. 2006. Regression of an esophageal ulcer using a dietary supplement containing melatonin. *J Pineal Res* 40(4):355–6.

Ganguly, K., P. Kundu, A. Banerjee, R. J. Reiter, and S. Swarnakar. 2006. Hydrogen peroxide-mediated downregulation of matrix metalloprotease-2 in indomethacin-induced acute gastric ulceration is blocked by melatonin and other antioxidants. *Free Radic Biol Med* 41 (6):911–25.

Ham, M., and J. D. Kaunitz. 2007. Gastroduodenal defense. *Curr Opin Gastroenterol* 23 (6):607–16.

Jaworek, J., T. Brzozowski, and S. J. Konturek. 2005. Melatonin as an organoprotector in the stomach and the pancreas. *J Pineal Res* 38 (2):73–83.

Kato, K., S. Asai, I. Murai, T. Nagata, Y. Takahashi, S. Komuro, A. Iwasaki, K. Ishikawa, and Y. Arakawa. 2001. Melatonin's gastroprotective and antistress roles involve both central and peripheral effects. *J Gastroenterol* 36 (2):91–5.

Klupinska, G., C. Chojnacki, A. Harasiuk, A. Stepien, P. Wichan, K. Stec-Michalska, and J. Chojnacki. 2006. [Nocturnal secretion of melatonin in subjects with asymptomatic and symptomatic *Helicobacter pylori* infection]. *Pol Merkur Lekarski* 21 (123):239–42.

Klupinska, G., M. Wisniewska-Jarosinska, A. Harasiuk, C. Chojnacki, K. Stec-Michalska, J. Blasiak, R. J. Reiter, and J. Chojnacki. 2006. Nocturnal secretion of melatonin in patients with upper digestive tract disorders. *J Physiol Pharmacol* 57 Suppl 5:41–50.

Komarov, F. I., S. I. Rappoport, N. K. Malinovskaia, L. A. Voznesenskaia, and L. Vetterberg. 2003. [Melatonin: ulcer disease and seasons of the year]. *Klin Med (Mosk)* 81 (9):17–21.

Malinovskaya, N., F. I. Komarov, S. I. Rapoport, L. A. Voznesenskaya, and L. Wetterberg. 2001. Melatonin production in patients with duodenal ulcer. *Neuro Endocrinol Lett* 22 (2):109–17.

Malinovskaia, N. K., F. I. Komarova, S. I. Rapoport, N. T. Raikhlin, I. M. Kvetnoi, A. A. Lakshin, L. A. Voznesenskaia, and M. I. Rasulov. 2006.

[Melatonin in treatment of duodenal ulcer]. *Klin Med (Mosk)* 84 (1):5–11.

Malinovskaia, N. K., S. I. Rapoport, N. I. Zherna-kova, S. N. Rybnikova, L. I. Postnikova, and I. E. Parkhomenko. 2007. [Antihelicobacter effects of melatonin]. *Klin Med (Mosk)* 85 (3):40–3.

Osadchuk, M. A., and AIu Kulidzhanov. 2005. [Melanin-producing and NO-synthase gastric cells and the processes of cell regeneration in gastric and duodenal ulcers]. *Klin Med (Mosk)* 83 (9):34–7.

Reiter, R. J., D. X. Tan, J. C. Mayo, R. M. Sainz, J. Leon, and D. Bandyopadhyay. 2003. Neurally-mediated and neurally-independent beneficial actions of melatonin in the gastrointestinal tract. *J Physiol Pharmacol* 54 Suppl 4:113–25.

Rapoport, S. I., N. T. Raikhlin, N. K. Malinovskaia, and A. A. Lakshin. 2003. [Ultrastructural changes in cells of the antral gastric mucosa in patients with duodenal ulcers treated with melatonin]. *Ter Arkh* 75 (2):10–4.

Sener, G., F. O. Goren, N. B. Ulusoy, Y. Ersoy, S. Arbak, and G. A. Dulger. 2005. Protective effect of melatonin and omeprazole against alen-dronat-induced gastric damage. *Dig Dis Sci* 50 (8):1506–12.

Singh, P., V. K. Bhargava, and S. K. Garg. 2002. Effect of melatonin and beta-carotene on indo-methacin induced gastric mucosal injury. *Indian J Physiol Pharmacol* 46 (2):229–34.

Turcan, M., A. Iacobovici, and I. Haulica. 1997. [Melatonin and ubiquinone as endogenous antioxidant factors]. *Rev Med Chir Soc Med Nat Iasi* 101 (1–2):92–7.

Fujita, T., and K. Sakurai. 1995. Efficacy of glutamine-enriched enteral nutrition in an experimental model of mucosal ulcerative colitis. *Br J Surg* 82 (6):749–51.

Shive, W., R. N. Snider, B. Dubilier, J. C. Rude, G. E. Clark, Jr., and J. O. Ravel. 1957. Glutamine in treatment of peptic ulcer; preliminary report. *Tex State J Med* 53 (11):840–2.

van der Hulst, R. R. W. J. et al. 1993. Glutamine and the preservation of gut integrity. *Lancet* 341:1363–1365.

Ziegler, T. R., K. Benfell, R. J. Smith, L. S. Young, E. Brown, E. Ferrari-Baliviera, D. K. Lowe, and D. W. Wilmore. 1990. Safety and metabolic effects of L-glutamine administration in humans. *JPEN J Parenter Enteral Nutr* 14 (4 Suppl):137S–146S.

Hornsby-Lewis, L., M. Shike, P. Brown, M. Klang, D. Pearlstone, and M. F. Brennan. 1994. L-glutamine supplementation in home total parenteral nutrition patients: stability, safety, and effects on intestinal absorption. *JPEN J Parenter Enteral Nutr* 18 (3):268–73.

Gaby, A. R. 1996. The role of coenzyme Q10 in clinical medicine: Part I. *Alterna Med Rev* 1(1)11–17.

Cho, C. H., and C. W. Ogle. 1978. A correlative study of the antiulcer effects of zinc sulphate in stressed rats. *Eur J Pharmacol* 48 (1):97–105.

Frommer, D. J. 1975. The healing of gastric ulcers by zinc sulphate. *Med J Aust* 2 (21):793–6.

Oner, G., N. M. Bor, E. Onuk, and Z. N. Oner. 1981. The role of zinc ion in the development of gastric ulcers in rats. *Eur J Pharmacol* 70 (2):241–3.

Vattem, D. A., R. Ghaedian, and K. Shetty. 2005. Enhancing health benefits of berries through phenolic antioxidant enrichment: focus on cranberry. *Asia Pac J Clin Nutr* 14 (2):120–30.

Burger, O., E. Weiss, N. Sharon, M. Tabak, I. Neeman, and I. Ofek. 2002. Inhibition of *Helicobacter pylori* adhesion to human gastric mucus by a high-molecular-weight constituent of cranberry juice. *Crit Rev Food Sci Nutr* 42 (3 Suppl):279–84.

Zhang, L., J. Ma, K. Pan, V. L. Go, J. Chen, and W. C. You. 2005. Efficacy of cranberry juice on *Helicobacter pylori* infection: a double-blind, randomized placebo-controlled trial. *Helicobacter* 10 (2):139–45.

Shmuely, H., J. Yahav, Z. Samra, G. Chodick, R. Koren, Y. Niv, and I. Ofek. 2007. Effect of cranberry juice on eradication of *Helicobacter pylori* in patients treated with antibiotics and a proton pump inhibitor. *Mol Nutr Food Res* 51 (6):746–51.

Additional Medical Conditions that Might be Indirectly Linked to Low Stomach Acid

67 Gloor, M., K. Heinkel, and U. Schulz. 1972. [Gastric function tests in patients with acne vulgaris, rosacea and rosacea-like perioral dermatitis]. *Z Haut Geschlechtskr* 47 (7):267–71.

Schulz, U., and R. Drunkenmolle. 1971. [Correlations between disorders of gastric secretion and skin diseases]. *Z Gesamte Inn Med* 26 (9):Suppl:112 c.

68 Wright, J. Autoimmune Disorders: A General Approach. Unpublished paper.

69 Wright, J. and L. Lenard. *Why Stomach Acid Is Good For You: Natural Relief For Heartburn, Indigestion, and GERD* (New York: M. Evans & Company, Inc., 2001), 41.

70 Faulkner-Hogg, K. B., W. S. Selby, and R. H. Loblay. 1999. Dietary analysis in symptomatic patients with coeliac disease on a gluten-free diet: the role of trace amounts of gluten and non-gluten food intolerances. *Scand J Gastroenterol* 34 (8):784–9.

Karnam, U. S., L. R. Felder, and J. B. Raskin. 2004. Prevalence of occult celiac disease in patients with iron-deficiency anemia: a prospective study. *South Med J* 97 (1):30–4.

71 Bray, G. 1931. The hypochlorhydria of asthma in childhood. *Quarterly J Med*, 24:181–197.

72 Wright, J. and L. Lenard. *Why Stomach Acid Is Good For You: Natural Relief For Heartburn, Indigestion, and GERD* (New York: M. Evans & Company, Inc., 2001), 41.

73 Alonso, N., M. L. Granada, I. Salinas, A. M. Lucas, J. L. Reverter, J. Junca, A. Oriol, and A. Sanmarti. 2005. Serum pepsinogen I: an early marker of pernicious anemia in patients with type 1 diabetes. *J Clin Endocrinol Metab* 90 (9):5254–8.

Rabinowitch, I. M. 1949. Achlorhydria and its clinical significance in diabetes mellitus. *Am J Dig Dis* 16 (9):322–32.

74 Schulz, U., and R. Drunkenmolle. 1971. [Correlations between disorders of gastric secretion and skin diseases]. *Z Gesamte Inn Med* 26 (9):Suppl:112 c.

75 Fravel, R. 1920. The occurrence of hypochlorhydria in gall-bladder disease. *Am J Med* 159:512–517.

76 Kuiunen, P., A. Kuusi, and J. Maenpaa. 1980. Gastric findings in adolescents treated for Graves' disease. *Acta Paediatr Scand* 69 (4):535–6.

Watatani, Y., and N. Aoki. 1984. [Changes of gastrin levels in autoimmune thyroid disorders. Part I: Thyroid functions and gastrin levels]. *Nippon Naibunpi Gakkai Zasshi* 60 (3):171–82.

Wiersinga, W. M., and J. L. Touber. 1980. The relation between gastrin, gastric acid and thyroid function disorders. *Acta Endocrinol (Copenh)* 95 (3):341–9.

77 Wright, J. and L. Lenard. *Why Stomach Acid Is Good For You: Natural Relief For Heartburn, Indigestion, and GERD* (New York: M. Evans & Company, Inc., 2001), 41

78 Andreani, G., and C. Bagni. 1950. [Research on gastric function in multiple sclerosis.]. *Riv Patol Nerv Ment* 71 (3):475–83.

Lenský, P. 1968. Altered gastric acidity in patients with multiple sclerosis. *Cesk Gastroenterol Vyz* (8):526–30.

Rettig, K., and U. Rettig. 1960. [Acid relationships and intestinal bacteria in the gastric juice in multiple sclerosis.]. *Psychiatr Neurol Med Psychol (Leipz)* 12:90–4.

Soeder, M., and E. Kahl. 1955. [Disorders of the gastric acid secretion in multiple sclerosis.]. *Nervenarzt* 26 (2):79–80.

79 Wright, J. Autoimmune Disorders: A General Approach. Unpublished paper.

80 Hayes, D. M., J. F. Martin, and T. F. O'Brien, Jr. 1970. Pernicious anemia with atrophic gastritis in a 17 year old boy. *South Med J* 63 (4):429–31.

Howitz, J., and M. Schwartz. 1971. Vitiligo, achlorhydria, and pernicious anaemia. *Lancet* 1 (7713):1331–4.

Lanzon-Miller, S., R. E. Pounder, M. R. Hamilton, N. A. Chronos, S. Ball, J. E. Mercieca, M. Olausson, and C. Cederberg. 1987. Twenty-four-hour intragastric acidity and plasma gastrin concentration in healthy subjects and patients with duodenal or gastric ulcer, or pernicious anaemia. *Aliment Pharmacol Ther* 1 (3):225–37.

Xiao, S. D., S. J. Jiang, Y. Shi, D. Z. Zhang, Y. B. Hu, W. Z. Liu, and J. M. Yuan. 1990. Pernicious anemia and type A atrophic gastritis in the Chinese. *Chin Med J (Engl)* 103 (3):192–6.

81 Wright, J. Autoimmune Disorders: A General Approach. Unpublished paper.

82 Wright, J. Results of Heidelberg gastric analysis by radiotelemetry. Personal communication.

83 Edström, G. 1939. Magensejrerion und Grundumsatz bei den chronischen rheumatischen Arthritiden. *Acta Med Scand* 99:228–256.

Henriksson, K., K. Uvnas-Moberg, C. E. Nord, C. Johansson, and R. Gullberg. 1986. Gastrin, gastric acid secretion, and gastric microflora in patients with rheumatoid arthritis. *Ann Rheum Dis* 45 (6):475–83.

Lucchesi, O., and M. Lucchesi. 1945. Gastric acidity and rheumatoid arthritis. *Gastroenterology* 5:299–302.

Marcolongo, R., P. F. Bayeli, and M. Montagnani. 1979. Gastrointestinal involvement in rheumatoid arthritis: A biopsy study. *J Rheumatol* 6:163–173.

Rooney, P. J., W. C. Dick, R. C. Imrie, D. Turner, K. D. Buchanan, and J. Ardill. 1978. On the relationship between gastrin, gastric secretion, and adjuvant arthritis in rats. *Ann Rheum Dis* 37 (5):432–5.

Rowden, D. R., I. L. Taylor, J. A. Richter, R. S. Pinals, and R. A. Levine. 1978. Is hypergastrinaemia associated with rheumatoid arthritis? *Gut* 19 (11):1064–7.

Woodwark, A., and R. Wallis. 1912. The relation of the gastric secretion to rheumatoid arthritis. *Lancet*, October 5, 942–945.

84 Gough, A., D. Andrews, P. A. Bacon, and P. Emery. 1995. Evidence of omeprazole-induced small bowel bacterial overgrowth in patients with scleroderma. *Br J Rheumatol* 34 (10):976–7.

85 Pokorny, G., G. Karacsony, J. Lonovics, J. Hudak, J. Nemeth, and V. Varro. 1991. Types of atrophic gastritis in patients with primary Sjogren's syndrome. *Ann Rheum Dis* 50 (2):97–100.

Sugaya, T., H. Sakai, T. Sugiyama, and K. Imai. 1995. [Atrophic gastritis in Sjogren's syndrome]. *Nippon Rinsho* 53 (10):2540–4.

86 Wright, J. and L. Lenard. *Why Stomach Acid Is Good For You: Natural Relief For Heartburn, Indigestion, and GERD* (New York: M. Evans & Company, Inc., 2001), 41.

87 Howitz, J., and M. Schwartz. 1971. Vitiligo, achlorhydria, and pernicious anaemia. *Lancet* 1 (7713):1331–4.

Zauli, D., A. Tosti, G. Biasco, F. Miserocchi, A. Patrizi, D. Azzaroni, G. Andriani, G. Di Febo, and C. Callegari. 1986. Prevalence of autoimmune atrophic gastritis in vitiligo. *Digestion* 34 (3):169–72.

Side Effects of Prescription-Strength Antacids

88 http://www.astrazeneca-us.com/pi/Nexium.pdf and http://www.astrazeneca-us.com/pi/Prilosec.pdf (accessed January 14, 2008).

89 Ho, P. M., T. M. Maddox, L. Wang, S. D. Fihn, R. L. Jesse, E. D. Peterson, and J. S. Rumsfeld. Risk of adverse outcomes associated with concomitant use of clopidogrel and proton pump inhibitors following acute coronary syndrome. *JAMA* 301(9): 937-944.

The Alternative Approach to Stomach Problems

90 Hart A. Apple Cider Vinegar and Getting Rid of Heartburn. http://ezinearticles.com/?Apple-Cider-Vinegar-and-Getting-Rid-of-Heartburn&id=533799 (accessed January 14, 2008).

91 Henry, E. B., A. Carswell, A. Wirz, V. Fyffe, and K. E. McColl. 2005. Proton pump inhibitors reduce

the bioavailability of dietary vitamin C. *Aliment Pharmacol Ther* 22 (6):539–45.

92 Giri, R. K., T. Parija, and B. R. Das. 1999. d-limonene chemoprevention of hepatocarcinogenesis in AKR mice: inhibition of c-jun and c-myc. *Oncol Rep* 6 (5):1123–7.

Kawamori, T., T. Tanaka, Y. Hirose, M. Ohnishi, and H. Mori. 1996. Inhibitory effects of d-limonene on the development of colonic aberrant crypt foci induced by azoxymethane in F344 rats. *Carcinogenesis* 17 (2):369–72.

Nakaizumi, A., M. Baba, H. Uehara, H. Iishi, and M. Tatsuta. 1997. d-Limonene inhibits N-nitrosobis(2-oxopropyl)amine induced hamster pancreatic carcinogenesis. *Cancer Lett* 117 (1):99–103.

Uedo, N., M. Tatsuta, H. Iishi, M. Baba, N. Sakai, H. Yano, and T. Otani. 1999. Inhibition by D-limonene of gastric carcinogenesis induced by N-methyl-N'-nitro-N-nitrosoguanidine in Wistar rats. *Cancer Lett* 137 (2):131–6.

Willette, R. C., L. Barrow, R. Doster , J. Wilkins, J. S. Wilkins, and J. P. Heggers. Purified d-limonene: an effective agent for the relief of occasional symptoms of heartburn. Proprietary study. WRC Laboratories, Inc. Galveston, TX.

Yano, H., M. Tatsuta, H. Iishi, M. Baba, N. Sakai, and N. Uedo. 1999. Attenuation by d-limonene of sodium chloride-enhanced gastric carcinogenesis induced by N-methyl-N'-nitro-N-nitrosoguanidine in Wistar rats. *Int J Cancer* 82 (5):665–8.

93 Pereira Rde, S. 2006. Regression of gastroesopha-
    geal reflux disease symptoms using dietary sup-
    plementation with melatonin, vitamins and ami-
    noacids: comparison with omeprazole. *J Pineal
    Res* 41 (3):195–200.

94 Werbach, M. R. 2008. Melatonin for the treatment
    of gastroesophageal reflux disease. *Altern Ther
    Health Med* 14 (4):54–8.

Bibliography

Antacids

Studies on Long-Term Use and on Adverse Effects

AstraZeneca. Prilosec Prescribing Information. http://www.astrazeneca-us.com/pi/Prilosec.pdf (accessed January 14, 2008).

Boustani, M., K. S. Hall, K. A. Lane, H. Aljadhey, S. Gao, F. Unverzagt, M. D. Murray, A. Ogunniyi, and H. Hendrie. 2007. The association between cognition and histamine-2 receptor antagonists in African Americans. *J Am Geriatr Soc* 55 (8):1248–53.

Brunner, G., W. Creutzfeldt, U. Harke, and R. Lamberts. 1988. Therapy with omeprazole in patients with peptic ulcerations resistant to extended high-dose ranitidine treatment. *Digestion* 39 (2):80–90.

Colin-Jones, D. G., M. J. Langman, D. H. Lawson, and M. P. Vessey. 1983. Postmarketing surveillance of the safety of cimetidine: 12 month mortality report. *Br Med J (Clin Res Ed)* 286 (6379):1713–6.

Dial, S., K. Alrasadi, C. Manoukian, A. Huang, and D. Menzies. 2004. Risk of Clostridium difficile diarrhea among hospital inpatients prescribed proton pump inhibitors: cohort and case-control studies. *CMAJ* 171 (1):33–8.

Dial, S., J. A. Delaney, A. N. Barkun, and S. Suissa. 2005. Use of gastric acid-suppressive agents and the risk of community-acquired Clostridium difficile-associated disease. *JAMA* 294 (23):2989–95.

Dial, S., J. A. Delaney, V. Schneider, and S. Suissa. 2006. Proton pump inhibitor use and risk of community-acquired Clostridium difficile-associated disease defined by prescription for oral vancomycin therapy. *CMAJ* 175 (7):745–8.

Fried, M., H. Siegrist, R. Frei, F. Froehlich, P. Duroux, J. Thorens, A. Blum, J. Bille, J. J. Gonvers, and K. Gyr. 1994. Duodenal bacterial overgrowth during treatment in outpatients with omeprazole. *Gut* 35 (1):23–6.

Galbraith, R. A., and J. J. Michnovicz. 1989. The effects of cimetidine on the oxidative metabolism of estradiol. *N Engl J Med* 321 (5):269–74.

Garcia Rodríguez, L. A., and A. Ruigómez. 1997. Gastric acid, acid-suppressing drugs, and bacterial gastroenteritis: how much of a risk? This study, based on ever-users (any antacid, any dosage and duration) of acid-suppressing drugs, minimized the danger of bacterial gastroenteritis. *Epidemiology* 8 (5):571–4.

Garcia Rodriguez, L. A., J. Lagergren, and M. Lindblad. 2006. Gastric acid suppression and risk of oesophageal and gastric adenocarcinoma: a nested case control study in the UK. *Gut* 55 (11):1538–44.

Goddard, A. F., and R. C. Spiller. 1996. The effect of omeprazole on gastric juice viscosity, pH and bacterial counts. *Aliment Pharmacol Ther* 10 (1):105–9.

Gough, A., D. Andrews, P. A. Bacon, and P. Emery. 1995. Evidence of omeprazole-induced small bowel bacterial overgrowth in patients with scleroderma. *Br J Rheumatol* 34 (10):976–7.

Gulmez, S. E., A. Holm, H. Frederiksen, T. G. Jensen, C. Pedersen, and J. Hallas. 2007. Use of proton pump inhibitors and the risk of community-acquired pneumonia: a population-based case-control study. *Arch Intern Med* 167 (9):950–5.

Health Sciences Institute. *Preventing Esophageal Cancer.* http://www.hsibaltimore.com/ealerts/ea200503/ea20050315.html (accessed January 11, 2008).

Heatley, R. V., and G. M. Sobala. 1993. Acid suppression and the gastric flora. *Baillieres Clin Gastroenterol* 7 (1):167–81.

Herzog, P., and K. H. Holtermuller. 1982. Antacid therapy—changes in mineral metabolism. *Scand J Gastroenterol Suppl* 75:56–62.

Howenstine, J. 2004. The Health Risks of Blocking Acid Production by the Stomach. http://www.newswithviews.com/howenstine/james21.html (accessed June 3, 2007).

Hurwitz, A., and D. L. Schlozman. 1974. Effects of antacids on gastrointestinal absorption of isoniazid in rat and man. *Am Rev Respir Dis* 109 (1):41–7.

Hutchinson, S., and R. Logan. 1997. The effect of long-term omeprazole on the glucose-hydrogen breath test in elderly patients. *Age Ageing* 26 (2):87–9.

Insogna, K. L., D. R. Bordley, J. F. Caro, and D. H. Lockwood. 1980. Osteomalacia and weakness from excessive antacid ingestion. *JAMA* 244 (22):2544–6.

Kaehnv, W. D. et al. 1977. Gastrointestinal absorption of aluminum from aluminum-containing antacids. *New Engl J Med* 296:1389–90.

Howenstine J. The Health Risks of Blocking Acid Production by the Stomach. December 9, 2004. http://www.newswithviews.com/howenstine/james21.htm. Accessed June 3, 2007.

Jansen, J. B., E. C. Klinkenberg-Knol, S. G. Meuwissen, J. W. De Bruijne, H. P. Festen, P. Snel, A. E. Luckers, I. Biemond, and C. B. Lamers. 1990. Effect of long-term treatment with omeprazole on serum gastrin and serum group A and C pepsinogens in patients with reflux esophagitis. *Gastroenterology* 99 (3):621–8.

Karmeli, Y., R. Stalnikowitz, R. Eliakim, and G. Rahav. 1995. Conventional dose of omeprazole alters gastric flora. *Dig Dis Sci* 40 (9):2070–3.

Koop, H. 1992. Review article: metabolic consequences of long-term inhibition of acid secretion by omeprazole. *Aliment Pharmacol Ther* 6 (4):399–406.

Koop, H., M. Klein, and R. Arnold. 1990. Serum gastrin levels during long-term omeprazole treatment. *Aliment Pharmacol Ther* 4 (2):131–8.

Koop, H., C. Naumann-Koch, and R. Arnold. 1990. Effect of omeprazole on serum gastrin levels: influence of age and sex. *Z Gastroenterol* 28 (11):603–5.

Kraus, A., and L. F. Flores-Suarez. 1995. Acute gout associated with omeprazole. *Lancet* 345 (8947):461–2.

Kuipers, E. J., L. Lundell, E. C. Klinkenberg-Knol, N. Havu, H. P. Festen, B. Liedman, C. B. Lamers, J. B. Jansen, J. Dalenback, P. Snel, G. F. Nelis, and S. G. Meuwissen. 1996. Atrophic gastritis and *Helicobacter pylori* infection in patients with reflux esophagitis treated with omeprazole or fundoplication. *N Engl J Med* 334 (16):1018–22.

Kuipers, E. J., A. M. Uyterlinde, A. S. Pena, H. J. Hazenberg, E. Bloemena, J. Lindeman, E. C. Klinkenberg-Knol, and S. G. Meuwissen. 1995. Increase of *Helicobacter pylori*-associated corpus gastritis during acid suppressive therapy: implications for long-term safety. *Am J Gastroenterol* 90 (9):1401–6.

Laheij, R. J., M. C. Sturkenboom, R. J. Hassing, J. Dieleman, B. H. Stricker, and J. B. Jansen. 2004. Risk of community-acquired pneumonia and use of gastric acid-suppressive drugs. *JAMA* 292 (16):1955–60.

Laheij, R. J., M. C. Van Ijzendoorn, M. J. Janssen, and J. B. Jansen. 2003. Gastric acid-suppressive therapy and community-acquired respiratory infections. *Aliment Pharmacol Ther* 18 (8):847–51.

Lamberts, R., W. Creutzfeldt, F. Stockmann, U. Jacubaschke, S. Maas, and G. Brunner. 1988. Long-term omeprazole treatment in man: effects on gastric endocrine cell populations. *Digestion* 39 (2):126–35.

Lamberts, R., W. Creutzfeldt, H. G. Struber, G. Brunner, and E. Solcia. 1993. Long-term omeprazole therapy in peptic ulcer disease: gastrin, endocrine cell growth, and gastritis. *Gastroenterology* 104 (5):1356–70.

Lewis, S. J., S. Franco, G. Young, and S. J. O'Keefe. 1996. Altered bowel function and duodenal bacterial overgrowth in patients treated with omeprazole. *Aliment Pharmacol Ther* 10 (4):557–61.

Lindquist, M., and I. R. Edwards. 1992. Endocrine adverse effects of omeprazole. *BMJ* 305 (6851):451–2.

Logan, R. P., M. M. Walker, J. J. Misiewicz, P. A. Gummett, Q. N. Karim, and J. H. Baron. 1995. Changes in the intragastric distribution of *Helicobacter pylori* during treatment with omeprazole. *Gut* 36 (1):12–6.

National Heartburn Alliance. Get Heartburn Smart. http://www.heartburnalliance.org/pdfs/brochure.pdf (accessed December 10, 2007).

Nitschmann, S. 2006. [Increased risk of pneumonia through gastric acid reduction. Partial evaluation of the Integrated Primary Care Information Project (IPCIP)]. *Internist (Berl)* 47 (4):441–2; discussion 442.

O'Connor, H. J. 1999. Review article: *Helicobacter pylori* and gastro-oesophageal reflux disease-clinical implications and management. *Aliment Pharmacol Ther* 13 (2):117–27.

O'Neil-Cutting, M. A., and W. H. Crosby. 1986. The effect of antacids on the absorption of simultaneously ingested iron. *JAMA* 255 (11):1468–70.

Patel, T. A., P. Abraham, V. J. Ashar, S. J. Bhatia, and P. S. Anklesaria. 1995. Gastric bacterial overgrowth accompanies profound acid suppression. *Indian J Gastroenterol* 14 (4):134–6.

Pereira, S. P., N. Gainsborough, and R. H. Dowling. 1998. Drug-induced hypochlorhydria causes high duodenal bacterial counts in the elderly. *Aliment Pharmacol Ther* 12 (1):99–104.

Piper, D. W. 1995. A comparative overview of the adverse effects of antiulcer drugs. *Drug Saf* 12 (2):120–38.

Pounder, R., and J. Smith. 1990. Drug-induced changes of plasma gastrin concentration. *Gastroenterol Clin North Am* 19 (1):141–53.

Reinke, C. M., J. Breitkreutz, and H. Leuenberger. 2003. Aluminium in over-the-counter drugs: risks outweigh benefits? *Drug Saf* 26 (14):1011–25.

Ricci, R. M., and K. C. Deering. 1996. Erythema nodosum caused by omeprazole. *Cutis* 57 (6):434.

Robertson, D. J., H. Larsson, S. Friis, L. Pedersen, J. A. Baron, and H. T. Sorensen. 2007. Proton pump inhibitor use and risk of colorectal cancer: a population-based, case-control study. *Gastroenterology* 133 (3):755–60.

Saadeh, G., T. Bauer, A. Licata, and L. Sheeler. 1987. Antacid-induced osteomalacia. *Cleve Clin J Med* 54 (3):214–6.

Saltzman, J. R., J. A. Kemp, B. B. Golner, M. C. Pedrosa, G. E. Dallal, and R. M. Russell. 1994. Effect of hypochlorhydria due to omeprazole treatment or atrophic gastritis on protein-bound vitamin B12 absorption. *J Am Coll Nutr* 13 (6):584–91.

Sataloff, R. T. 2005. Community-acquired pneumonia and use of gastric acid-suppressive drugs. *JAMA* 293 (7):795–6; author reply 796.

Shindo, K., M. Machida, M. Fukumura, K. Koide, and R. Yamazaki. 1998. Omeprazole induces altered bile acid metabolism. *Gut* 42 (2):266–71.

Solcia, E., G. Rindi, N. Havu, and G. Elm. 1989. Qualitative studies of gastric endocrine cells in patients treated long-term with omeprazole. *Scand J Gastroenterol Suppl* 166:129–37; discussion 138–9.

Spencer, H., and L. Kramer. 1985. Osteoporosis: calcium, fluoride, and aluminum interactions. *J Am Coll Nutr* 4 (1):121–8.

Spencer, H., L. Kramer, C. Norris, and D. Osis. 1982. Effect of small doses of aluminum-containing antacids on calcium and phosphorus metabolism. *Am J Clin Nutr* 36 (1):32–40.

Spencer, H., and M. Lender. 1979. Adverse effects of aluminum-containing antacids on mineral metabolism. *Gastroenterology* 76 (3):603–6.

Steinberg, W. M., C. E. King, and P. P. Toskes. 1980. Malabsorption of protein-bound cobalamin but not unbound cobalamin during cimetidine administration. *Dig Dis Sci* 25 (3):188–91.

Sturniolo, G. C., M. C. Montino, L. Rossetto, A. Martin, R. D'Inca, A. D'Odorico, and R. Naccarato. 1991. Inhibition of gastric acid secretion reduces zinc absorption in man. *J Am Coll Nutr* 10 (4):372–5.

Teichtahl, H., I. J. Kronborg, N. D. Yeomans, and P. Robinson. 1996. Adult asthma and gastro-oesophageal reflux: the effects of omeprazole therapy on asthma. *Aust N Z J Med* 26 (5):671–6.

Theisen, J., D. Nehra, D. Citron, J. Johansson, J. A. Hagen, P. F. Crookes, S. R. DeMeester, C. G. Bremner, T. R. DeMeester, and J. H. Peters. 2000. Suppression of gastric acid secretion in patients with gastroesophageal reflux disease results in gastric bacterial overgrowth and deconjugation of bile acids. *J Gastrointest Surg* 4 (1):50–4.

Vagnini, F., and B. Fox. 2006. Preventing pharmaceutical-induced nutritional deficiencies. *Life Extension,* March:72–9.

Vanpee, D., E. Delgrange, J. B. Gillet, and J. Donckier. 2000. Ingestion of antacid tablets (Rennie) and acute confusion. *J Emerg Med* 19 (2):169–71.

Waldum, H. L., E. Brenna, P. M. Kleveland, A. K. Sandvik, and U. Syversen. 1993. Review article: the use of gastric acid-inhibitory drugs—physiological and pathophysiological considerations. *Aliment Pharmacol Ther* 7 (6):589–96.

Weberg, R., A. Berstad, J. Aaseth, and J. A. Falch. 1985. Mineral-metabolic side effects of low-dose antacids. *Scand J Gastroenterol* 20 (6):741–6.

Zavros, Y., G. Rieder, A. Ferguson, L. C. Samuelson, and J. L. Merchant. 2002. Genetic or chemical hypochlorhydria is associated with inflammation that modulates parietal and G-cell populations in mice. *Gastroenterology* 122 (1):119–33.

Antacids

Other Articles and Studies

AstraZeneca. Nexium Prescribing Information. http://www.astrazeneca-us.com/pi/Nexium.pdf (accessed January 14, 2008).

Claessens, A. A., E. R. Heerdink, C. B. Lamers, J. T. van Eijk, and H. G. Leufkens. 2001. Factors associated with non-response in proton pump inhibitor users: a study of lansoprazole therapy. Pharm World Sci 23 (3):107–10.

Horwich, L., and R. Galloway. 1965. Treatment of gastric ulceration with carbenoxolone sodium: clinical and radiological evaluation. *Br Med J* 2 (5473):1274–7.

Lewis, J. R. 1974. Carbenoxolone sodium in the treatment of peptic ulcer. A review. *JAMA* 229 (4):460–2.

Mayo Clinic Health Letter. 2006. If stomach acid helps digest food, how is food digested if you take an antacid after a meal? Mayo Clin Health Lett 24(3):8.

Morgan, A. G., W. A. McAdam, C. Pacsoo, and A. Darnborough. 1982. Comparison between cimetidine and Caved-S in the treatment of gastric ulceration, and subsequent maintenance therapy. *Gut* 23 (6):545–51.

Morgan, A. G., W. A. McAdam, C. Pacsoo, B. E. Walker, and A. V. Simmons. 1978. Cimetidine: an advance in gastric ulcer treatment? *Br Med J* 2 (6148):1323–6.

Tanner, L., Digestion Treatments Soar For Kids, Associated Press. October 7, 2007, http://www.jsonline.com/story/index.aspx?id=671539 (accessed November 7, 2007).

Low Stomach Acid

Associated Issues and Diseases

Allison, J. R. 1945. The relation of hydrochloric acid and vitamin B complex deficiency in certain skin diseases. In this study of vitamin B-deficient patients with skin disorders, nearly all had low stomach acid. Vitamin B complex combined with hydrochloric acid was a more successful treatment than treatment that used only vitamin B. *South Med J* 38:235.

Alonso, N., M. L. Granada, I. Salinas, A. M. Lucas, J. L. Reverter, J. Junca, A. Oriol, and A. Sanmarti. 2005. Serum pepsinogen I: an early marker of pernicious anemia in patients with type 1 diabetes. *J Clin Endocrinol Metab* 90 (9):5254–8.

Andreani, G., and C. Bagni. 1950. [Research on gastric function in multiple sclerosis.]. *Riv Patol Nerv Ment* 71 (3):475–83.

Baik, H. W., and R. M. Russell. 1999. Vitamin B12 deficiency in the elderly. *Annu Rev Nutr* 19:357–77.

Berg, R. D. 1981. The translocation of normal flora bacteria from the gastrointestinal tract to the mesenteric lymph nodes and other organs. Review. *Microecology, Therapy* 11:27–34.

Berg, R. D., E. Wommack, and E. A. Deitch. 1988. Immunosuppression and intestinal bacterial overgrowth synergistically promote bacterial translocation. *Arch Surg* 123 (11):1359–64.

Bezwoda, W., R. Charlton, T. Bothwell, J. Torrance, and F. Mayet. 1978. The importance of gastric hydrochloric acid in the absorption of nonheme food iron. *J Lab Clin Med* 92 (1):108–16.

Bloomfield, A., and W. Polland. Anacidity with cancer of the stomach. *Gastric Anacidity: Its Relation to Disease* (New York: MacMillan, 1933), 125–136.

Bo-Linn, G. W., G. R. Davis, D. J. Buddrus, S. G. Morawski, C. Santa Ana, and J. S. Fordtran. 1984. An evaluation of the importance of gastric acid secretion in the absorption of dietary calcium. *J Clin Invest* 73 (3):640–7.

Bray, G. 1931. The hypochlorhydria of asthma in childhood. *Quarterly J Med* 24:181–197.

Breneman, J. C. 1968. Allergy elimination diet as the most effective gallbladder diet. *Ann Allergy* 26 (2):83–7.

Brownie, S. 2006. Why are elderly individuals at risk of nutritional deficiency? *Int J Nurs Pract* 12 (2):110–8.

Brummer, R. J., and R. W. Stockbrugger. 1996. Effect of nizatidine 300 mg at night and omeprazole 20 mg in the morning on 24-hour intragastric pH and bacterial overgrowth in patients with acute duodenal ulcer. *Dig Dis Sci* 41 (10):2048–54.

Buckley, C. 1996. Pityriasis rosea-like eruption in a patient receiving omeprazole. *Br J Dermatol* 135 (4):660–1.

Canani, R. B., P. Cirillo, P. Roggero, C. Romano, B. Malamisura, G. Terrin, A. Passariello, F. Manguso, L. Morelli, and A. Guarino. 2006. Therapy with gastric acidity inhibitors increases the risk of acute gastroenteritis and community-acquired pneumonia in children. *Pediatrics* 117 (5):e817–20.

Capper, W. M., T. J. Butler, J. O. Kilby, and M. J. Gibson. 1967. Gallstones, gastric secretion, and flatulent dyspepsia. *Lancet* 1 (7487):413–5.

Carey, J., and M. Wetherby. 1941. Gastric observations in achlorhydria. *J Dig Dis*. 8:401–407.

Champagne, E. T. 1988. Effects of pH on mineral-phytate, protein-mineral-phytate, and mineral-fiber interactions. Possible consequences of atrophic gastritis on mineral bioavailability from high-fiber foods. *J Am Coll Nutr* 7 (6):499–508.

Champagne, E., Possible consequences of reduced gastric acid secretion on mineral bioavailability from high-fiber diets, in *Chronic Gastritis and Hypochlorhydria in the Elderly*, ed. P. Holt and R. Russell, 171–186 (Boca Raton, FL: CRC Press, 1993).

Christiansen, P. M. 1968. The incidence of achlorhydria and hypochlorhydria in healthy subjects and patients with gastrointestinal diseases. *Scand J Gastroenterol* 3 (5):497–508.

Clemons, T. E., R. C. Milton, R. Klein, J. M. Seddon, and F. L. Ferris, 3rd. 2005. Risk factors for the incidence of Advanced Age-Related Macular Degeneration in the Age-Related Eye Disease Study (AREDS) AREDS report no. 19. *Ophthalmology* 112 (4):533–9.

Colorado State University. Pathophysiology of the Digestive System. http://arbl.cvmbs.colostate.edu/hbooks/pathphys/digestion (accessed February 29, 2008).

Creutzfeldt, W., and R. Lamberts. 1991. Is hypergastrinaemia dangerous to man? *Scand J Gastroenterol Suppl* 180:179–91.

Dotevall, G., and A. Walan. 1969. Gastric secretion of acid and intrinsic factor in patients with hyper- and hypothyroidism. *Acta Med Scand* 186 (6):529–33.

Douglas, I. J., C. Cook, U. Chakravarthy, R. Hubbard, A. E. Fletcher, and L. Smeeth. 2007. A case-control study of drug risk factors for age-related macular degeneration. *Ophthalmology* 114 (6):1164–9.

Driks, M. R., D. E. Craven, B. R. Celli, M. Manning, R. A. Burke, G. M. Garvin, L. M. Kunches, H. W. Farber, S. A. Wedel, and W. R. McCabe. 1987. Nosocomial pneumonia in intubated patients given sucralfate as compared with antacids or histamine type 2 blockers. The role of gastric colonization. *N Engl J Med* 317 (22):1376–82.

Edström, G. 1939. Magensejrerion und Grundumsatz bei den chronischen rheumatischen Arthritiden. This study correlates low stomach acid with chronic arthritis. *Acta Med Scand* 99:228–256.

Ekenved, G., L. Halvorsen, and L. Solvell. 1976. Influence of a liquid antacid on the absorption of different iron salts. *Scand J Haematol Suppl* 28:65–77.

Faulkner-Hogg, K. B., W. S. Selby, and R. H. Loblay. 1999. Dietary analysis in symptomatic patients with coeliac disease on a gluten-free diet: the role of trace amounts of gluten and non-gluten food intolerances. *Scand J Gastroenterol* 34 (8):784–9.

Federico, M. 2005. Does treating gastroesophageal reflux cause pneumonia? *J Pediatr Gastroenterol Nutr* 40 (3):386–7.

Fiorino, A. S. 1996. Hypercalcemia and alkalosis due to the milk-alkali syndrome: a case report and review. *Yale J Biol Med* 69 (6):517–23.

Fox, J. G., and T. C. Wang. 2007. Inflammation, atrophy, and gastric cancer. *J Clin Invest* 117 (1):60–9.

Fravel, R. 1920. The occurrence of hypochlorhydria in gall-bladder disease. *Am J Med* 159:512–517.

Freston, J. W., K. Borch, S. J. Brand, E. Carlsson, W. Creutzfeldt, R. Hakanson, L. Olbe, E. Solcia, J. H. Walsh, and M. M. Wolfe. 1995. Effects of hypochlorhydria and hypergastrinemia on structure and function of gastrointestinal cells. A review and analysis. *Dig Dis Sci* 40 (2 Suppl):50S–62S.

George, S., and J. D. Clark. 2000. Milk alkali syndrome-an unusual syndrome causing an unusual complication. *Postgrad Med J* 76 (897):422–3.

Gitelson, S. 1971. Gastrectomy, achlorhydria and cholera. *Isr J Med Sci* 7 (5):663–7.

Gledhill, T., R. J. Leicester, B. Addis, N. Lightfoot, J. Barnard, N. Viney, D. Darkin, and R. H. Hunt. 1985. Epidemic hypochlorhydria. *Br Med J (Clin Res Ed)* 290 (6479):1383–6.

Goldin, B., and S. Gorbach, Bacterial overgrowth in atrophic gastritis in *Chronic Gastritis and Hypochlorhydria in the Elderly*, ed. P. Holt and R. Russell, 143–156 (Boca Raton, FL: CRC Press, 1993).

Gregor, J. C. 2004. Acid suppression and pneumonia: a clinical indication for rational prescribing. *JAMA* 292 (16):2012–3.

Guslandi, M., A. Pellegrini, and M. Sorghi. 1999. Gastric mucosal defences in the elderly. *Gerontology* 45 (4):206–8.

Hartung, E., and O. Steinbrocker. 1935. Gastric acidity in chronic arthritis. *Ann Intern Med.* 9:252–257.

Hayes, D. M., J. F. Martin, and T. F. O'Brien, Jr. 1970. Pernicious anemia with atrophic gastritis in a 17 year old boy. *South Med J* 63 (4):429–31.

Henderson, L. M., G. J. Brewer, J. B. Dressman, S. Z. Swidan, D. J. DuRoss, C. H. Adair, J. L. Barnett, and R. R. Berardi. 1995. Effect of intragastric pH on the absorption of oral zinc acetate and zinc oxide in young healthy volunteers. *JPEN J Parenter Enteral Nutr* 19 (5):393–7.

Henriksson, K., K. Uvnas-Moberg, C. E. Nord, C. Johansson, and R. Gullberg. 1986. Gastrin, gastric acid secretion, and gastric microflora in patients with rheumatoid arthritis. *Ann Rheum Dis* 45 (6):475–83.

Hicklin, J. et al. 1980. The effect of diet in rheumatoid arthritis. *Clin Allergy.* 10:463.

Howden, C. W., and R. H. Hunt. 1987. Relationship between gastric secretion and infection. *Gut* 28 (1):96–107.

Howitz, J., and M. Schwartz. 1971. Vitiligo, achlorhydria, and pernicious anaemia. *Lancet* 1 (7713):1331–4.

Ivanovich, P., H. Fellows, and C. Rich. 1967. The absorption of calcium carbonate. *Ann Intern Med* 66 (5):917–23.

Jacobs, A., J. H. Lawrie, C. C. Entwistle, and H. Campbell. 1966. Gastric acid secretion in chronic iron-deficiency anaemia. *Lancet* 2 (7456):190–2.

Jacobs, P., T. Bothwell, and R. W. Charlton. 1964. Role of Hydrochloric Acid in Iron Absorption. *J Appl Physiol* 19:187–8.

Karnam, U. S., L. R. Felder, and J. B. Raskin. 2004. Prevalence of occult celiac disease in patients with iron-deficiency anemia: a prospective study. *South Med J* 97 (1):30–4.

Kassarjian, Z., and R. M. Russell. 1989. Hypochlorhydria: a factor in nutrition. *Annu Rev Nutr* 9:271–85.

Keuter, E. J. W. 1959. Deficiency of vitamin B complex, presenting itself psychiatrically as an atypical, endogenous depression. *Nutr Abstr Rev* 29:273 (Abstract).

King, C. E., J. Leibach, and P. P. Toskes. 1979. Clinically significant vitamin B12 deficiency secondary to malabsorption of protein-bound vitamin B12. *Dig Dis Sci* 24 (5):397–402.

Knowles, F., and H. Decker. 1926. Gastric acidity and acne vulgaris. *Arch Dermatol Syphilology* 13:215–218.

Kuiunen, P., A. Kuusi, and J. Maenpaa. 1980. Gastric findings in adolescents treated for Graves' disease. *Acta Paediatr Scand* 69 (4):535–6.

Kunz, L. J., and W. R. Waddell. 1956. Association of Salmonella enteritis with operations on the stomach. *N Engl J Med* 255 (12):555–9.

Kuster, G. G., W. H. ReMine, and M. B. Dockerty. 1972. Gastric cancer in pernicious anemia and in patients with and without achlorhydria. *Ann Surg* 175 (5):783–9.

Lanzon-Miller, S., R. E. Pounder, M. R. Hamilton, S. Ball, N. A. Chronos, F. Raymond, M. Olausson, and C. Cederberg. 1987. Twenty-four-hour intragastric acidity and plasma gastrin concentration before and during treatment with either ranitidine or omeprazole. *Aliment Pharmacol Ther* 1 (3):239–51.

Lanzon-Miller, S., R. E. Pounder, M. R. Hamilton, N. A. Chronos, S. Ball, J. E. Mercieca, M. Olausson, and C. Cederberg. 1987. Twenty-four-hour intragastric acidity and plasma gastrin concentration in healthy subjects and patients with duodenal or gastric ulcer, or pernicious anaemia. *Aliment Pharmacol Ther* 1 (3):225–37.

Lazlo, J., Effect of gastrointestinal conditions on the mineral-binding properties of dietary fibers, in *Mineral Absorption in the Monogastric GI Tract (Advances in Experimental Medicine and Biology, Vol. 249)*, ed. F. Dintzis and J. Lazlo (New York: Plenum Press, 1993).

Lensky, P. 1968. [Altered gastric acidity in patients with multiple sclerosis]. *Cesk Gastroenterol Vyz* 22 (8):526–30.

Lichtman, S. N., J. Wang, R. B. Sartor, C. Zhang, D. Bender, F. G. Dalldorf, and J. H. Schwab. 1995. Reactivation of arthritis induced by small bowel bacterial overgrowth in rats: role of cytokines, bacteria, and bacterial polymers. *Infect Immun* 63 (6):2295–301.

Lucarelli, S., G. Corrado, A. Pelliccia, G. D'Ambrini, M. Cavaliere, M. Barbato, D. Lendvai, and T. Frediani. 2000. Cyclic vomiting syndrome and food allergy/intolerance in seven children: a possible association. *Eur J Pediatr* 159 (5):360–3.

Lucchesi, O., and M. Lucchesi. 1945. Gastric acidity and rheumatoid arthritis. *Gastroenterology* 5:299–302.

Lyman, H. M. 1897. Chronic catarrhal gastritis. *JAMA* 28(8):439–442.

Maltby, E. J. 1934. The Digestion of Beef Proteins in the Human Stomach. *J Clin Invest* 13 (2):193–207.

Marcolongo, R., P. F. Bayeli, and M. Montagnani. 1979. Gastrointestinal involvement in rheumatoid arthritis: a biopsy study. *J Rheumatol* 6 (2):163–73.

Marcuard, S. P., L. Albernaz, and P. G. Khazanie. 1994. Omeprazole therapy causes malabsorption of cyanocobalamin (vitamin B12). *Ann Intern Med* 120 (3):211–5.

McCarthy, C. F. 1976. Nutritional defects in patients with malabsorption. *Proc Nutr Soc* 35 (1):37–40.

Morgan, J. E., C. W. Kaiser, W. Johnson, W. G. Doos, Y. Dayal, L. Berman, and D. Nabseth. 1983. Gastric carcinoid (gastrinoma) associated with achlorhydria (pernicious anemia). *Cancer* 51 (12):2332–40.

Morley, J. E. 2007. The aging gut: physiology. *Clin Geriatr Med* 23 (4):757–67, v–vi.

Murray, M. J., and N. Stein. 1968. A gastric factor promoting iron absorption. *Lancet* 1 (7543):614–6.

Nalin, D. R., R. J. Levine, M. M. Levine, D. Hoover, E. Bergquist, J. McLaughlin, J. Libonati, J. Alam, and R. B. Hornick. 1978. Cholera, non-vibrio cholera, and stomach acid. *Lancet* 2 (8095):856–9.

Ogilvie, J. 1935. The gastric secretion in anaemia. *Arch Dis Childhood* 10:143–148.

Pedrosa, M., and R. Russell, Folate and vitamin B12 absorption in atrophic gastritis, in *Chronic Gastritis and Hypochlorhydria in the Elderly*, ed. P. Holt and R. Russell, 157–169 (Boca Raton, FL: CRC Press, 1993).

Peura, D., and R. Guerrant, Achlorhydria and enteric bacteria infections, in *Chronic Gastritis and Hypochlorhydria in the Elderly*, ed. P. Holt and R. Russell, 127–142 (Boca Raton, FL: CRC Press, 1993).

Pokorny, G., G. Karacsony, J. Lonovics, J. Hudak, J. Nemeth, and V. Varro. 1991. Types of atrophic gastritis in patients with primary Sjogren's syndrome. *Ann Rheum Dis* 50 (2):97–100.

Rabinowitch, I. M. 1949. Achlorhydria and its clinical significance in diabetes mellitus. *Am J Dig Dis* 16 (9):322–32.

Recker, R. R. 1985. Calcium absorption and achlorhydria. *N Engl J Med* 313 (2):70–3.

Rettig, K., and U. Rettig. 1960. [Acid relationships and intestinal bacteria in the gastric juice in multiple sclerosis.]. *Psychiatr Neurol Med Psychol (Leipz)* 12:90–4.

Reunala, T., and P. Collin. 1997. Diseases associated with dermatitis herpetiformis. *Br J Dermatol* 136 (3):315–8.

Rooney, P. J., W. C. Dick, R. C. Imrie, D. Turner, K. D. Buchanan, and J. Ardill. 1978. On the relationship between gastrin, gastric secretion, and adjuvant arthritis in rats. *Ann Rheum Dis* 37 (5):432–5.

Rowden, D. R., I. L. Taylor, J. A. Richter, R. S. Pinals, and R. A. Levine. 1978. Is hypergastrinaemia associated with rheumatoid arthritis? *Gut* 19 (11):1064–7.

Russell, R. M., B. B. Golner, S. D. Krasinski, J. A. Sadowski, P. M. Suter, and C. L. Braun. 1988. Effect of antacid and H2 receptor antagonists on the intestinal absorption of folic acid. *J Lab Clin Med* 112 (4):458–63.

Saltzman, J. R., K. V. Kowdley, M. C. Pedrosa, T. Sepe, B. Golner, G. Perrone, and R. M. Russell. 1994. Bacterial overgrowth without clinical malabsorption in elderly hypochlorhydric subjects. *Gastroenterology* 106 (3):615–23.

Schulz, U., and R. Drunkenmolle. 1971. [Correlations between disorders of gastric secretion and skin diseases]. *Z Gesamte Inn Med* 26 (9):Suppl:112 c.

Segal, H. L., and I. M. Samloff. 1973. Gastric cancer—increased frequency in patients with achlorhydria. *Am J Dig Dis* 18 (4):295–9.

Simon, S. W. 1951. Vitamin B12 therapy in allergy and chronic dermatoses. *J Allergy* 22 (2):183–5.

Sipponen, P., F. Laxen, K. Huotari, and M. Harkonen. 2003. Prevalence of low vitamin B12 and high homocysteine in serum in an elderly male population: association with atrophic gastritis and *Helicobacter pylori* infection. *Scand J Gastroenterol* 38 (12):1209–16.

Skikne, B. S., S. R. Lynch, and J. D. Cook. 1981. Role of gastric acid in food iron absorption. *Gastroenterology* 81 (6):1068–71.

Soeder, M., and E. Kahl. 1955. [Disorders of the gastric acid secretion in multiple sclerosis.]. *Nervenarzt* 26 (2):79–80.

Spivacke, C., and M. Golob. 1942. Depression of hydrochloric acid secretion in allergic conditions. *Rev Gastroenterol* 9:376–379.

Sugaya, T., H. Sakai, T. Sugiyama, and K. Imai. 1995. [Atrophic gastritis in Sjogren's syndrome]. *Nippon Rinsho* 53 (10):2540–4.

Svendsen, J. H., C. Dahl, L. B. Svendsen, and P. M. Christiansen. 1986. Gastric cancer risk in achlorhydric patients. A long-term follow-up study. *Scand J Gastroenterol* 21 (1):16–20.

Tedesco, A. S., and P. J. Lynch. 1979. Association of dermatitis herpetiformis and pernicious anemia. *Arch Dermatol* 115 (9):1117.

van de Laar, M. A, and J. K. van der Korst. 1992. Food intolerance in rheumatoid arthritis. A double blind controlled trial of the clinical effects of elimination of milk allergens and azo dyes. *Ann Rheum Dis* 51:298–302.

Van Loon, F. P., J. D. Clemens, M. Shahrier, D. A. Sack, C. B. Stephensen, M. R. Khan, G. H. Rabbani, M. R. Rao, and A. K. Banik. 1990. Low gastric acid as a risk factor for cholera transmission: application of a new non-invasive gastric acid field test. *J Clin Epidemiol* 43 (12):1361–7.

Watatani, Y., and N. Aoki. 1984. [Changes of gastrin levels in autoimmune thyroid disorders. Part I: Thyroid functions and gastrin levels]. *Nippon Naibunpi Gakkai Zasshi* 60 (3):171–82.

Wetzel, N. C., W. C. Fargo et al. 1949. Growth failure in school children as associated with vitamin B12 deficiency; response to oral therapy. *Science* 110 (2868):651–3.

Wiersinga, W. M., and J. L. Touber. 1980. The relation between gastrin, gastric acid and thyroid function disorders. *Acta Endocrinol (Copenh)* 95 (3):341–9.

Wood, R., and C. Serfaty-Lacrosniere, Effects of gastric acidity and atrophic gastritis on calcium and zinc absorption in humans, in *Chronic Gastritis and Hypochlorhydria in the Elderly*, ed. P. Holt and R. Russell, 187–204 (Boca Raton, FL: CRC Press, 1993).

Woodwark, A., and R. Wallis. 1912. The relation of the gastric secretion to rheumatoid arthritis. *Lancet* October 5:942–945.

Wright, J. Results of Heidelberg gastric analysis by radiotelemetry. Unpublished.

Wright, J. Autoimmune Disorders: A General Approach. Unpublished paper.

Xiao, S. D., S. J. Jiang, Y. Shi, D. Z. Zhang, Y. B. Hu, W. Z. Liu, and J. M. Yuan. 1990. Pernicious anemia and type A atrophic gastritis in the Chinese. *Chin Med J (Engl)* 103 (3):192–6.

Yang, Y. X., J. D. Lewis, S. Epstein, and D. C. Metz. 2006. Long-term proton pump inhibitor therapy and risk of hip fracture. *JAMA* 296 (24):2947–53.

Zauli, D., A. Tosti, G. Biasco, F. Miserocchi, A. Patrizi, D. Azzaroni, G. Andriani, G. Di Febo, and C. Callegari. 1986. Prevalence of autoimmune atrophic gastritis in vitiligo. *Digestion* 34 (3):169–72.

Low Stomach Acid

Other Articles

Cedars Sinai Website. http://healthinfo.cedars-sinai .edu/library/healthguide/en-us/IllnessConditions/ topic.asp? hwid=hw99177 (accessed June 23, 2006). Also cited in *Life Extension, Collectors' Edition 2007*.

Saltzman, J., Epidemiology and natural history of atrophic gastritis, in *Chronic Gastritis and Hypochlorhydria in the Elderly*, ed. P. Holt and R. Russell, 31–48 (Boca Raton, FL: CRC Press, 1993).

Sharp, G. S., and H. W. Fisher. 1967. The diagnosis and treatment of achlorhydria: ten-year study. *J Am Geriatr Soc* 15:786.

H. pylori: Associations with Ulcers, Low Stomach Acid, Gastric Cancer, and Other Problems

An international association between *Helicobacter pylori* infection and gastric cancer. The EUROGAST Study Group. 1993. *Lancet* 341 (8857):1359–62.

Argent, R. H., R. J. Thomas, F. Aviles-Jimenez, D. P. Letley, M. C. Limb, E. M. El-Omar, and J. C. Atherton. 2008. Toxigenic *Helicobacter pylori* infection precedes gastric hypochlorhydria in cancer relatives, and *H. pylori* virulence evolves in these families. *Clin Cancer Res* 14 (7):2227–35.

Australian Institute of Policy and Science. Barry Marshall: Gastroenterologist. http://www.tallpoppies .net.au/cavalcade/marshall.html (accessed September 9, 2006).

Baker, B. *H. pylori* suggested as possible underlying factor in rosacea. *Skin & Allergy News* September 1994, 4.

Bayerdorffer, E., A. Neubauer, B. Rudolph, C. Thiede, N. Lehn, S. Eidt, and M. Stolte. 1995. Regression of primary gastric lymphoma of mucosa-associated lymphoid tissue type after cure of *Helicobacter pylori* infection. MALT Lymphoma Study Group. *Lancet* 345 (8965):1591–4.

Blaser, M. J. 1996. The bacteria behind ulcers. *Sci Am* 274 (2):104–7.

Borody, T., Noonan T., P. Cole et al. 1989. Triple therapy of *H. pylori* can reverse hypochlorhydria. *Am J Gastroenterology* 96:A53.

Calvert, R., J. Randerson, P. Evans, L. Cawkwell, F. Lewis, M. F. Dixon, A. Jack, R. Owen, C. Shiach, and G. J. Morgan. 1995. Genetic abnormalities during transition from Helicobacter-pylori-associated gastritis to low-grade MALToma. *Lancet* 345 (8941):26–7.

Cater, R. E., 2nd. 1992. The clinical importance of hypochlorhydria (a consequence of chronic Helicobacter infection): its possible etiological role in mineral and amino acid malabsorption, depression, and other syndromes. *Med Hypotheses* 39 (4):375–83.

———. 1992. Helicobacter (aka Campylobacter) pylori as the major causal factor in chronic hypochlorhydria. *Med Hypotheses* 39 (4):367–74.

Das, U. N. 1998. Hypothesis: cis-unsaturated fatty acids as potential anti-peptic ulcer drugs. *Prostaglandins Leukot Essent Fatty Acids* 58 (5):377–80.

De Koster, E., M. Buset, E. Fernandes et al. 1994. *Helicobacter pylori*: the link with gastric cancer. *Europ J Cancer Prev* 3(3):247–257.

D'Elios, M. M., C. Montecucco, and M. de Bernard. 2007. VacA and HP-NAP, Ying and Yang of *Helicobacter pylori*-associated gastric inflammation. *Clin Chim Acta* 381 (1):32–8.

Fendrick, A. M., M. E. Chernew, R. A. Hirth, B. S. Bloom, R. R. Bandekar, and J. M. Scheiman. 1999. Clinical and economic effects of population-based *Helicobacter pylori* screening to prevent gastric cancer. *Arch Intern Med* 159 (2):142–8.

Forman, D., D. G. Newell, F. Fullerton, J. W. Yarnell, A. R. Stacey, N. Wald, and F. Sitas. 1991. Association between infection with *Helicobacter pylori* and risk of gastric cancer: evidence from a prospective investigation. *BMJ* 302 (6788):1302–5.

Gotz, J. M., J. L. Thio, H. W. Verspaget, G. J. Offerhaus, I. Biemond, C. B. Lamers, and R. A. Veenendaal. 1997. Treatment of *Helicobacter pylori* infection favourably affects gastric mucosal superoxide dismutases. *Gut* 40 (5):591–6.

Gotz, J. M., C. I. van Kan, H. W. Verspaget, I. Biemond, C. B. Lamers, and R. A. Veenendaal. 1996. Gastric mucosal superoxide dismutases in *Helicobacter pylori* infection. *Gut* 38 (4):502–6.

Gross, H., N. Freundich, and H. Dawley, Is cancer a contagious disease: No, *Business Week*, July 14, 1997, 70–76.

Hansson, L. E., O. Nyren, A. W. Hsing, R. Bergstrom, S. Josefsson, W. H. Chow, J. F. Fraumeni, Jr., and H. O. Adami. 1996. The risk of stomach cancer in patients with gastric or duodenal ulcer disease. *N Engl J Med* 335 (4):242–9.

Henschel, E., G. Brandstatter, B. Dragosics et al. 1993. Effect of ranitidine and amoxicillin plus metronidazole on the eradication of Helcobacter pylori and the recurrence of duodenal ulcer. *New Engl J Med* 328:308–312.

Hood, H. M., C. Wark, P. A. Burgess, D. Nicewander, and M. W. Scott. 1999. Screening for *Helicobacter pylori* and nonsteroidal anti-inflammatory drug use in medicare patients hospitalized with peptic ulcer disease. *Arch Intern Med* 159 (2):149–54.

Hwang, H., J. Dwyer, and R. M. Russell. 1994. Diet, *Helicobacter pylori* infection, food preservation and gastric cancer risk: are there new roles for preventative factors? *Nutr Rev* 52 (3):75–83.

Iijima, K., H. Sekine, T. Koike, A. Imatani, S. Ohara, and T. Shimosegawa. 2004. Long-term effect of *Helicobacter pylori* eradication on the reversibility of acid secretion in profound hypochlorhydria. *Aliment Pharmacol Ther* 19 (11):1181–8.

Kuipers, E. J., A. Lee, E. C. Klinkenberg-Knol, and S. G. Meuwissen. 1995. Review article: the development of atrophic gastritis—*Helicobacter pylori* and the effects of acid suppressive therapy. *Aliment Pharmacol Ther* 9 (4):331–40.

Kuipers, E. J., A. S. Pena, and S. G. Meuwissen. 1995. [*Helicobacter pylori* infection as causal factor in the development of carcinoma and lymphoma of the stomach; report WHO consensus conference]. *Ned Tijdschr Geneeskd* 139 (14):709–12.

Kuipers, E. J., J. C. Thijs, and H. P. Festen. 1995. The prevalence of *Helicobacter pylori* in peptic ulcer disease. *Aliment Pharmacol Ther* 9 Suppl 2:59–69.

Kuipers, E. J., A. M. Uyterlinde, A. S. Pena, R. Roosendaal, G. Pals, G. F. Nelis, H. P. Festen, and S. G. Meuwissen. 1995. Long-term sequelae of *Helicobacter pylori* gastritis. *Lancet* 345 (8964):1525–8.

Lai, L. H., and J. J. Sung. 2007. *Helicobacter pylori* and benign upper digestive disease. *Best Pract Res Clin Gastroenterol* 21 (2):261–79.

Lochhead, P., and E. M. El-Omar. 2007. *Helicobacter pylori* infection and gastric cancer. *Best Pract Res Clin Gastroenterol* 21 (2):281–97.

Marshall, B. J., and J. R. Warren. 1984. Unidentified curved bacilli in the stomach of patients with gastritis and peptic ulceration. *Lancet* 1 (8390):1311–5.

Marshall, B.J. Unidentified curved bacillus on gastric epithelium in active chronic gastritis. *Lancet* 1 (8336):1273–1275.

McColl, K., L. Murray, E. El-Omar, A. Dickson, A. El-Nujumi, A. Wirz, A. Kelman, C. Penny, R. Knill-Jones, and T. Hilditch. 1998. Symptomatic benefit from eradicating *Helicobacter pylori* infection in patients with nonulcer dyspepsia. *N Engl J Med* 339 (26):1869–74.

Mertz, H., *Helicobacter pylori*: Its role in gastritis, achlorhydria, and gastric carcinoma, in *Chronic Gastritis and Hypochlorhydria in the Elderly*, ed. P. Holt and R. Russell, 69–82 (Boca. Raton, FL: CRC Press, 1993).

Modena, J. L., G. O. Acrani, A. F. Micas, M. Castro, W. D. Silveira, R. B. Oliveira, and M. Brocchi. 2007. Correlation between *Helicobacter pylori* infection, gastric diseases and life habits among patients treated at a university hospital in Southeast Brazil. *Braz J Infect Dis* 11 (1):89–95.

Munoz, N. 1994. Is *Helicobacter pylori* a cause of gastric cancer? An appraisal of the seroepidemiological evidence. *Cancer Epidemiol Biomarkers Prev* 3 (5):445–51.

Murakami, K., M. Kodama, and T. Fujioka. 2006. Latest insights into the effects of *Helicobacter pylori* infection on gastric carcinogenesis. *World J Gastroenterol* 12 (17):2713–20.

Noguchi, K., K. Kato, T. Moriya, T. Suzuki, M. Saito, T. Kikuchi, J. Yang, A. Imatani, H. Sekine, S. Ohara, T. Toyota, T. Shimosegawa, and H. Sasano. 2002. Analysis of cell damage in *Helicobacter pylori*-associated gastritis. *Pathol Int* 52 (2):110–8.

Nomura, A., G. N. Stemmermann, P. H. Chyou, I. Kato, G. I. Perez-Perez, and M. J. Blaser. 1991. *Helicobacter pylori* infection and gastric carcinoma among Japanese Americans in Hawaii. *N Engl J Med* 325 (16):1132–6.

Parsonnet, J., G. D. Friedman, D. P. Vandersteen, Y. Chang, J. H. Vogelman, N. Orentreich, and R. K. Sibley. 1991. *Helicobacter pylori* infection and the risk of gastric carcinoma. *N Engl J Med* 325 (16):1127–31.

Riccardi, V. M., and J. I. Rotter. 1994. Familial *Helicobacter pylori* infection. Societal factors, human genetics, and bacterial genetics. *Ann Intern Med* 120 (12):1043–5.

Robinson, K., R. H. Argent, and J. C. Atherton. 2007. The inflammatory and immune response to *Helicobacter pylori* infection. *Best Pract Res Clin Gastroenterol* 21 (2):237–59.

Salih, B. A., M. F. Abasiyanik, N. Bayyurt, and E. Sander. 2007. H pylori infection and other risk factors associated with peptic ulcers in Turkish patients: a retrospective study. *World J Gastroenterol* 13 (23):3245–8.

Schubert, M. L. 2002. Gastric secretion. *Curr Opin Gastroenterol* 18 (6):639–49.

Slomiany, B. L., V. L. Murty, J. Piotrowski, and A. Slomiany. 1994. Gastroprotective agents in mucosal defense against *Helicobacter pylori*. *Gen Pharmacol* 25 (5):833–41.

Sobala, G. M., C. J. Schorah, B. Pignatelli, J. E. Crabtree, I. G. Martin, N. Scott, and P. Quirke. 1993. High gastric juice ascorbic acid concentrations in members of a gastric cancer family. *Carcinogenesis* 14 (2):291–2.

Sobala, G. M., C. J. Schorah, M. Sanderson, M. F. Dixon, D. S. Tompkins, P. Godwin, and A. T. Axon. 1989. Ascorbic acid in the human stomach. *Gastroenterology* 97 (2):357–63.

Suzuki, T., K. Matsuo, H. Ito, K. Hirose, K. Wakai, T. Saito, S. Sato, Y. Morishima, S. Nakamura, R. Ueda, and K. Tajima. 2006. A past history of gastric ulcers and *Helicobacter pylori* infection increase the risk of gastric malignant lymphoma. *Carcinogenesis* 27 (7):1391–7.

Szabo, S., X. Deng, T. Khomenko, L. Chen, G. Tolstanova, K. Osapay, Z. Sandor, and X. Xiong. 2007. New molecular mechanisms of duodenal ulceration. *Ann N Y Acad Sci* 1113:238–55.

Uemura, N., T. Mukai, S. Okamoto, S. Yamaguchi, H. Mashiba, K. Taniyama, N. Sasaki, K. Haruma, K. Sumii, and G. Kajiyama. 1997. Effect of *Helicobacter pylori* eradication on subsequent development of cancer after endoscopic resection of early gastric cancer. *Cancer Epidemiol Biomarkers Prev* 6 (8):639–42.

Wilson, K. T., and J. E. Crabtree. 2007. Immunology of *Helicobacter pylori*: insights into the failure of the immune response and perspectives on vaccine studies. *Gastroenterology* 133 (1):288–308.

Wotherspoon, A. C., C. Doglioni, T. C. Diss, L. Pan, A. Moschini, M. de Boni, and P. G. Isaacson. 1993. Regression of primary low-grade B-cell gastric lymphoma of mucosa-associated lymphoid tissue type after eradication of *Helicobacter pylori*. *Lancet* 342 (8871):575–7.

Xia, H. H., and N. J. Talley. 1998. *Helicobacter pylori* infection, reflux esophagitis, and atrophic gastritis: an unexplored triangle. *Am J Gastroenterol* 93 (3):394–400.

Zucca, E., F. Bertoni, E. Roggero, G. Bosshard, G. Cazzaniga, E. Pedrinis, A. Biondi, and F. Cavalli. 1998. Molecular analysis of the progression from *Helicobacter pylori*-associated chronic gastritis to mucosa-associated lymphoid-tissue lymphoma of the stomach. *N Engl J Med* 338 (12):804–10.

H. Pylori

Other Articles

Jancin, B. 1994. Pushing the *H. pylori* envelope: treat everyone with dyspepsia. *Family Practice News* 1:14.

Knipp, U., S. Birkholz, W. Kaup, and W. Opferkuch. 1993. Immune suppressive effects of *Helicobacter pylori* on human peripheral blood mononuclear cells. *Med Microbiol Immunol* 182 (2):63–76.

Noach, L. A., M. A. Bertola, M. P. Schwanz et al. 1994. Treatment of *Helicobacter pylori* infection and evaluation of various therapeutic trials. *Europ J Gastroenterol Hepatol* 6:585–591.

Parsonnet, J. 1996. *Helicobacter pylori* in the stomach— a paradox unmasked. *N Engl J Med* 335 (4):278–80.

Ulcers

Additional Articles

Andre, C., B. Moulinier, F. Andre, and S. Daniere. 1983. Evidence for anaphylactic reactions in peptic ulcer and varioliform gastritis. *Ann Allergy* 51 (2 Pt 2):325–8.

Kern, R.A., G. Stewart. 1931. Allergy in duodenal ulcer: incidence and significance of food hypersensitivities as observed in 32 patients. *J Allergy* 3:51.

Kumar, N., A. Kumar, S. L. Broor, J. O. Vij, and B. S. Anand. 1986. Effect of milk on patients with duodenal ulcers. *Br Med J (Clin Res Ed)* 293 (6548):666.

Salim, A. S. 1990. Oxygen-derived free radicals and the prevention of duodenal ulcer relapse: a new approach. *Am J Med Sci* 300 (1):1–6; discussion 7–8.

———. 1990. Removing oxygen-derived free radicals stimulates healing of ethanol-induced erosive gastritis in the rat. *Digestion* 47 (1):24–8.

———. 1993. The relationship between *Helicobacter pylori* and oxygen-derived free radicals in the mechanism of duodenal ulceration. *Intern Med* 32 (5):359–64.

Sanderson, C. R., and R. E. Davis. 1975. Serum pyridoxal in active peptic ulceration. *Gut* 16 (3):177–80.

Schumpelick, V., and E. Farthmann. 1976. [Study on the protective effect of vitamin A on stress ulcer of the rat (author's transl)]. *Arzneimittelforschung* 26 (3):386–8.

Siegel, J. 1974. Gastrointestinal ulcer—arthus reaction. *Ann Allergy* 32 (3):127–30.

———. 1977. Immunologic approach to the treatment and prevention of gastrointestinal ulcers. *Ann Allergy* 38 (1):27–41.

GERD

General Information

American Gastroenterological Association. Heartburn Facts. http://www.gastro.org/wmspage.cfm?parm1=467 (accessed January 11, 2008).

Bredenoord, A. J., A. Baron, and A. J. Smout. 2006. Symptomatic gastro-oesophageal reflux in a patient with achlorhydria. *Gut* 55 (7):1054–5.

Fass, R., and R. Dickman. 2006. Clinical consequences of silent gastroesophageal reflux disease. *Curr Gastroenterol Rep* 8 (3):195–201.

Gerd Information Resource Center. What is GERD? http://www.gerd.com/consumer/gerd.aspx (accessed January 14, 2008).

Havelund, T., and C. Aalykke. 1997. The efficacy of a pectin-based raft-forming anti-reflux agent in endoscopy-negative reflux disease. *Scand J Gastroenterol* 32 (8):773–7.

Havelund, T., C. Aalykke, and L. Rasmussen. 1997. Efficacy of a pectin-based anti-reflux agent on acid reflux and recurrence of symptoms and oesophagitis in gastro-oesophageal reflux disease. *Eur J Gastroenterol Hepatol* 9 (5):509–14.

Hill, D. J., R. G. Heine, D. J. Cameron, A. G. Catto-Smith, C. W. Chow, D. E. Francis, and C. S. Hosking. 2000. Role of food protein intolerance in infants with persistent distress attributed to reflux esopha-gitis. *J Pediatr* 136 (5):641–7.

Jacobson, B. C., S. C. Somers, C. S. Fuchs, C. P. Kelly, and C. A. Camargo, Jr. 2006. Body-mass index and symptoms of gastroesophageal reflux in women. *N Engl J Med* 354 (22):2340–8.

Maher, J. Common Indigestion: Millions of Americans Suffer From It. University of Iowa Health Science Relations. www.uihealthcare.com/topics/medicaldepartments/surgery/gerd/index.html (accessed October 29, 2007).

Maton, P., and M. Buron. 1991. Antacids revisited: A review of their clinical pharmacology and recommended therapeutic use. OTC antacids often carry drug interactions and side effects (especially in long term use). *Drugs* 57:855–870.

Maton, P. N. 2003. Profile and assessment of GERD pharmacotherapy. *Cleve Clin J Med* 70 Suppl 5:S51–70.

Mayo Clinic Website. Digestive System: Heartburn. http://www.mayoclinic.com/health/heartburn-gerd/DS00095 (accessed January 6, 2008).

National Institutes of Health. Your Digestive System and How It Works. http://digestive.niddk.nih.gov/ddiseases/pubs/yrdd (accessed January 6, 2008).

O'Connor, J. B., and J. E. Richter. 1998. Recognizing extraesophageal manifestations of GERD. *Intern Med* 19(10):40–48.

Prilosec OTC Website. What is the cause of heartburn? http://www.prilosecotc.com/heartburn/heartburncauses.jsp (accessed January 14, 2008).

Prilosec OTC Website. What does heartburn feel like? http://www.prilosecotc.com/heartburn/symptoms.jsp (accessed March 19, 2008).

Srinivasan, R., R. Tutuian, P. Schoenfeld, M. F. Vela, J. A. Castell, T. Isaac, I. Galaria, P. O. Katz, and D. O. Castell. 2004. Profile of GERD in the adult population of a northeast urban community. *J Clin Gastroenterol* 38 (8):651–7.

Waterhouse, E. T., C. Washington, and N. Washington. 2000. An investigation into the efficacy of the pectin based anti-reflux formulation-Aflurax. *Int J Pharm* 209 (1–2):79–85.

GERD

LES Pressure and Its Association with Level of Stomach Acid

Castell, D. O., and S. M. Levine. 1971. Lower esophageal sphincter response to gastric alkalinization. A new mechanism for treatment of heartburn with antacids. *Ann Intern Med* 74 (2):223–7.

Dent, J., and J. Hansky. 1976. Relationship of serum gastrin response to lower oesophageal sphincter pressure. *Gut* 17 (2):144–6.

Freeland, G. R., R. H. Higgs, and D. O. Castell. 1977. Lower esophageal sphincter response to oral administration of cimetidine in normal subjects. *Gastroenterology* 72 (1):28–30.

Higgs, R. H., R. D. Smyth, and D. O. Castell. 1974. Gastric alkalinization. Effect on lower-esophageal-sphincter pressure and serum gastrin. *N Engl J Med* 291 (10):486–90.

Kline, M. M., R. W. McCallum, N. Curry, and R. A. Sturdevant. 1975. Effect to gastric alkalinization on lower esophageal sphincter pressure and serum gastrin. *Gastroenterology* 68 (5 Pt 1):1137–9.

McCallum, R. W. 1985. Studies on the mechanism of the lower esophageal sphincter pressure response to alkali ingestion in humans. *Am J Gastroenterol* 80 (7):513–7.

Steinnon, O. A. The Longitudinal Muscle in Esophageal Disease, *Radiology Publishing,* May 1995, http://www.esophagushoncho.com (accessed March 17, 2008).

Wallin, L., T. Madsen, M. Brandsborg, O. Brandsborg, and N. E. Larsen. 1979. The influence of cimetidine on basal gastro-oesophageal sphincter pressure, intargastric pH, and serum gastrin concentration in normal subjects. *Scand J Gastroenterol* 14 (3):349–53.

GERD

Association with Cancer

Cohen, S., and H. P. Parkman. 1999. Heartburn—a serious symptom. *N Engl J Med* 340 (11):878–9.

Eckardt, V. F., G. Kanzler, and G. Bernhard. 2001. Life expectancy and cancer risk in patients with Barrett's esophagus: a prospective controlled investigation. *Am J Med* 111 (1):33–7.

El-Serag, H. B., E. J. Hepworth, P. Lee, and A. Sonnenberg. 2001. Gastroesophageal reflux disease is a risk factor for laryngeal and pharyngeal cancer. *Am J Gastroenterol* 96 (7):2013–8.

Garavello, W., E. Negri, R. Talamini, F. Levi, P. Zambon, L. Dal Maso, C. Bosetti, S. Franceschi, and C. La Vecchia. 2005. Family history of cancer, its combination with smoking and drinking, and risk of squamous cell carcinoma of the esophagus. *Cancer Epidemiol Biomarkers Prev* 14 (6):1390–3.

Kubo, A., T. R. Levin, G. Block, G. J. Rumore, C. P. Quesenberry, Jr., P. Buffler, and D. A. Corley. 2008. Dietary patterns and the risk of Barrett's esophagus. *Am J Epidemiol* 167 (7):839–46.

Lagergren, J., R. Bergstrom, A. Lindgren, and O. Nyren. 1999. Symptomatic gastroesophageal reflux as a risk factor for esophageal adenocarcinoma. *N Engl J Med* 340 (11):825–31.

Neegaard, L. Complications from Heartburn on the Rise, *Associated Press*, March 31, 2008. Source: American Cancer Society.

Williams, D. A. Healthy Diet Saves Your Throat, *Alternatives*, March 2008.

Dyspepsia

Azpiroz, F. Understanding Intestinal Gas. International Foundation for Functional Gastrointestinal Disorders. https://www.iffgd.org/store/downloadfile/214 (accessed January 4, 2008).

Eaton, K. K. 1992. Sugars in food intolerance and gut fermentation. *J Nutr Med* 3:295–301.

Hunnusett, A., J. Howard, and S. Davies. 1990. *Gut* fermentation (or the "auto-brewery" syndrome): a clinical test with initial observations and discussion. A simple test using measurements of blood alcohol levels (EtOH) may be useful in determining patients who ferment dietary carbohydrate in their gut. *J Nutr Med* 1:33–38.

Johannessen, T., H. Petersen, P. M. Kleveland, J. H. Dybdahl, A. K. Sandvik, E. Brenna, and H. Waldum. 1990. The predictive value of history in dyspepsia. *Scand J Gastroenterol* 25 (7):689–97.

Jones, R., and S. Lydeard. 1989. Prevalence of symptoms of dyspepsia in the community. *BMJ* 298 (6665):30–2.

Kaji, H., Y. Asanuma, O. Yahara, H. Shibue, M. Hisamura, N. Saito, Y. Kawakami, and M. Murao. 1984. Intragastrointestinal alcohol fermentation syndrome: report of two cases and review of the literature. *J Forensic Sci Soc* 24 (5):461–71.

Sanderson, C. R., and R. E. Davis. 1976. Serum pyridoxal in patients with gastric pathology. *Gut* 17 (5):371–4.

Aging and Its Effect on Gastric Function

Blechman, M. B., and A. M. Gelb. 1999. Aging and gastrointestinal physiology. *Clin Geriatr Med* 15 (3):429–38.

Geokas, M. C., and B. J. Haverback. 1969. The aging gastrointestinal tract. *Am J Surg* 117 (6):881–92.

Hosoda, S. 1992. The gastrointestinal tract and nutrition in the aging process: an overview. *Nutr Rev* 50 (12):372–3.

Krasinski, S. D., R. M. Russell, I. M. Samloff, R. A. Jacob, G. E. Dallal, R. B. McGandy, and S. C. Hartz. 1986. Fundic atrophic gastritis in an elderly population. Effect on hemoglobin and several serum nutritional indicators. *J Am Geriatr Soc* 34 (11):800–6.

Krentz, K., and H. Jablonowski, in *Gastrointestinal Tract Disorders in the Elderly*, ed. J. Hellemans, and G. Vantrappen (Edinburgh: Churchill Livingstone, 1984).

Lovat, L. B. 1996. Age related changes in gut physiology and nutritional status. *Gut* 38 (3):306–9.

Majumdar, A. P., R. Jaszewski, and M. A. Dubick. 1997. Effect of aging on the gastrointestinal tract and the pancreas. *Proc Soc Exp Biol Med* 215 (2):134–44.

Russell, R. M. 1992. Changes in gastrointestinal function attributed to aging. *Am J Clin Nutr* 55 (6 Suppl):1203S–1207S.

———. 1997. Gastric hypochlorhydria and achlorhydria in older adults. *JAMA* 278 (20):1659–60.

Natural Remedies for Stomach Disorders

Al-Habbal, M. J., Z. Al-Habbal, and F. U. Huwez. 1984. A double-blind controlled clinical trial of mastic and placebo in the treatment of duodenal ulcer. *Clin Exp Pharmacol Physiol* 11 (5):541–4.

Al-Said, M. S., A. M. Ageel, N. S. Parmar, and M. Tariq. 1986. Evaluation of mastic, a crude drug obtained from Pistacia lentiscus for gastric and duodenal anti-ulcer activity. *J Ethnopharmacol* 15 (3):271–8.

Aly, A. M., L. Al-Alousi, and H. A. Salem. 2005. Licorice: a possible anti-inflammatory and anti-ulcer drug. *AAPS PharmSciTech* 6 (1):E74–82.

Andersson, S., F. Barany, J. L. Caboclo, and T. Mizuno. 1971. Protective action of deglycyrrhizinized liquorice on the occurrence of stomach ulcers in pylorus-ligated rats. *Scand J Gastroenterol* 6 (8):683–6.

Anon. 2001. Picrorhiza kurroa. Monograph. *Altern Med Rev* 6(3):319–21.

Arakawa, T., H. Satoh, A. Nakamura, H. Nebiki, T. Fukuda, H. Sakuma, H. Nakamura, M. Ishikawa, M. Seiki, and K. Kobayashi. 1990. Effects of zinc L-carnosine on gastric mucosal and cell damage caused by ethanol in rats. Correlation with endogenous prostaglandin E2. *Dig Dis Sci* 35 (5):559–66.

Arora, A., and M. P. Sharma. 1990. Use of banana in non-ulcer dyspepsia. *Lancet* 335 (8689):612–3.

Baker, M. E. 1994. Licorice and enzymes other than 11 beta-hydroxysteroid dehydrogenase: an evolutionary perspective. *Steroids* 59 (2):136–41.

Bandyopadhyay, D., A. Bandyopadhyay, P. K. Das, and R. J. Reiter. 2002. Melatonin protects against gastric ulceration and increases the efficacy of ranitidine and omeprazole in reducing gastric damage. *J Pineal Res* 33 (1):1–7.

Bandyopadhyay, D., K. Biswas, M. Bhattacharyya, R. J. Reiter, and R. K. Banerjee. 2001. Gastric toxicity and mucosal ulceration induced by oxygen-derived reactive species: protection by melatonin. *Curr Mol Med* 1 (4):501–13.

Bandyopadhyay, D., and A. Chattopadhyay. 2006. Reactive oxygen species-induced gastric ulceration: protection by melatonin. *Curr Med Chem* 13 (10):1187–202.

Bandyopadhyay, D., G. Ghosh, A. Bandyopadhyay, and R. J. Reiter. 2004. Melatonin protects against piroxicam-induced gastric ulceration. *J Pineal Res* 36 (3):195–203.

Barbieri, S. S., V. Cavalca, S. Eligini, M. Brambilla, A. Caiani, E. Tremoli, and S. Colli. 2004. Apocynin prevents cyclooxygenase 2 expression in human monocytes through NADPH oxidase and glutathione redox-dependent mechanisms. *Free Radic Biol Med* 37 (2):156–65.

Bardhan, K. D., D. C. Cumberland, R. A. Dixon, and C. D. Holdsworth. 1978. Clinical trial of deglycyrrhizinised liquorice in gastric ulcer. *Gut* 19 (9):779–82.

Bennett, A., T. Clark-Wibberley, I. F. Stamford, and J. E. Wright. 1980. Aspirin-induced gastric mucosal damage in rats: cimetidine and deglycyrrhizinated liquorice together give greater protection than low doses of either drug alone. *J Pharm Pharmacol* 32 (2):151.

Bilici, D., H. Suleyman, Z. N. Banoglu, A. Kiziltunc, B. Avci, A. Ciftcioglu, and S. Bilici. 2002. Melatonin prevents ethanol-induced gastric mucosal damage possibly due to its antioxidant effect. *Dig Dis Sci* 47 (4):856–61.

Bone, K., Eleven things you can eat or drink to knock out the hidden factor behind chronic—even deadly—disease, *Nutrition & Healing*, March 2005, 8.

Bullock, C. 1984. Can plantains prevent ulcers? *Med Tribune* Nov. 28, 25(33):3.

Burger, O., E. Weiss, N. Sharon, M. Tabak, I. Neeman, and I. Ofek. 2002. Inhibition of *Helicobacter pylori* adhesion to human gastric mucus by a high-molecular-weight constituent of cranberry juice. *Crit Rev Food Sci Nutr* 42 (3 Suppl):279–84.

Chamberlin, D.T., and H. J. Perkin. 1938. The level of ascorbic acid in the blood and urine of patients with peptic ulcer. *Am J Dig Dis* 5:493.

Chander, R., N. K. Kapoor, and B. N. Dhawan. 1992. Effect of picroliv on glutathione metabolism in liver and brain of Mastomys natalensis infected with Plasmodium berghei. *Indian J Exp Biol* 30 (8):711–4.

Chander, R., K. Singh, P. K. Visen, N. K. Kapoor, and B. N. Dhawan. 1998. Picroliv prevents oxidation in serum lipoprotein lipids of Mastomys coucha infected with Plasmodium berghei. *Indian J Exp Biol* 36 (4):371–4.

Cheney, G. 1949. Rapid healing of peptic ulcers in patients receiving fresh cabbage juice. *Calif Med* 70 (1):10–5.

———. 1952. Vitamin U therapy of peptic ulcer. *Calif Med* 77 (4):248–52.

Cheney, G., S. H. Waxler, and I. J. Miller. 1956. Vitamin U therapy of peptic ulcer; experience at San Quentin Prison. *Calif Med* 84 (1):39–42.

Cho, C. H., W. M. Hui, B. W. Chen, C. T. Luk, and S. K. Lam. 1992. The cytoprotective effect of zinc L-carnosine on ethanol-induced gastric gland damage in rabbits. *J Pharm Pharmacol* 44 (4):364–5.

Cho, C. H., C. T. Luk, and C. W. Ogle. 1991. The membrane-stabilizing action of zinc carnosine (Z-103) in stress-induced gastric ulceration in rats. *Life Sci* 49 (23):PL189–94.

Cho, C. H., and C. W. Ogle. 1978. A correlative study of the antiulcer effects of zinc sulphate in stressed rats. *Eur J Pharmacol* 48 (1):97–105.

Das, S. K., V. Das, A. K. Gulati, and V. P. Singh. 1989. Deglycyrrhizinated liquorice in aphthous ulcers. *J Assoc Physicians India* 37 (10):647.

Dehpour, A. R., M. E. Zolfaghari, T. Samadian, and Y. Vahedi. 1994. The protective effect of liquorice components and their derivatives against gastric ulcer induced by aspirin in rats. *J Pharm Pharmacol* 46 (2):148–9.

de Souza Pereira, R. 2006. Regression of an esophageal ulcer using a dietary supplement containing melatonin. *J Pineal Res* 40(4):355–6.

Doll, R., and I. D. Hill. 1962. Triterpenoid liquorice compound in gastric and duodenal ulcer. *Lancet* 2 (7266):1166–7.

Doll, R., and F. Pygott. 1954. Clinical trial of Robaden and of cabbage juice in the treatment of gastric ulcer. *Lancet* 267 (6850):1200–4.

D'Souza, R. S., and V. G. Dhume. 1991. Gastric cytoprotection. *Indian J Physiol Pharmacol* 35 (2):88–98.

Englisch, W., C. Beckers, M. Unkauf, M. Ruepp, and V. Zinserling. 2000. Efficacy of Artichoke dry extract in patients with hyperlipoproteinemia. *Arzneimittelforschung* 50 (3):260–5.

Engqvist, A., F. von Feilitzen, E. Pyk, and H. Reich-ard. 1973. Double-blind trial of deglycyrrhizinated liquorice in gastric ulcer. *Gut* 14 (9):711–5.

Feldman, H., and T. Gilat. 1971. A trial of deglycyrrhi-zinated liquorice in the treatment of duodenal ulcer. *Gut* 12 (6):449–51.

Fishbein, L. et al. 1988. Fructo-oligosaccharides: a review. *Vet Hum Toxical* 30(2):104–107.

Frommer, D. J. 1975. The healing of gastric ulcers by zinc sulphate. *Med J Aust* 2 (21):793–6.

Fuhrman, B., S. Buch, J. Vaya, P. A. Belinky, R. Cole-man, T. Hayek, and M. Aviram. 1997. Licorice extract and its major polyphenol glabridin protect low-den-sity lipoprotein against lipid peroxidation: in vitro and ex vivo studies in humans and in atherosclerotic apolipoprotein E-deficient mice. *Am J Clin Nutr* 66 (2):267–75.

Fujita, T., and K. Sakurai. 1995. Efficacy of glutamine-enriched enteral nutrition in an experimental model of mucosal ulcerative colitis. *Br J Surg* 82 (6):749–51.

Fukai, T., A. Marumo, K. Kaitou, T. Kanda, S. Terada, and T. Nomura. 2002. Anti-*Helicobacter pylori* flavo-noids from licorice extract. *Life Sci* 71 (12):1449–63.

Furuta, S., S. Toyama, M. Miwa, T. Itabashi, H. Sano, and T. Yoneta. 1995. Residence time of polaprezinc (zinc L-carnosine complex) in the rat stomach and adhesiveness to ulcerous sites. *Jpn J Pharmacol* 67 (4):271–8.

Gaby, A.R. 1996. The role of coenzyme Q10 in clinical medicine: part I. *Alterna Med Rev* 1(1)11–17.

Galan, M. V., A. A. Kishan, and A. L. Silverman. 2004. Oral broccoli sprouts for the treatment of *Helicobacter pylori* infection: a preliminary report. *Dig Dis Sci* 49 (7–8):1088–90.

Ganguly, K., P. Kundu, A. Banerjee, R. J. Reiter, and S. Swarnakar. 2006. Hydrogen peroxide-mediated downregulation of matrix metalloprotease-2 in indomethacin-induced acute gastric ulceration is blocked by melatonin and other antioxidants. *Free Radic Biol Med* 41 (6):911–25.

Garcia-Plaza, A., J. I. Arenas, O. Belda, A. Diago, A. Dominguez, C. Fernandez, L. Martin, A. Pallares, L. Rodrigo, and J. de la Santa. 1996. [A multicenter clinical trial. Zinc acexamate versus famotidine in the treatment of acute duodenal ulcer. Study Group of Zinc acexamate (new UP doses)]. *Rev Esp Enferm Dig* 88 (11):757–62.

Gebhardt, R. 1997. Antioxidative and protective properties of extracts from leaves of the artichoke (Cynara scolymus L.) against hydroperoxide-induced oxidative stress in cultured rat hepatocytes. *Toxicol Appl Pharmacol* 144 (2):279–86.

Giri, R. K., T. Parija, and B. R. Das. 1999. d-limonene chemoprevention of hepatocarcinogenesis in AKR mice: inhibition of c-jun and c-myc. *Oncol Rep* 6 (5):1123–7.

Glavin, G. B. 1933. Ascorbic acid and cold restraint ulcer in rats: dose-response relationship. *Nutr Rep Int* 28:705.

Glick, L. 1982. Deglycyrrhizinated liquorice for peptic ulcer. *Lancet* 2 (8302):817.

Gotteland, M., O. Brunser, and S. Cruchet. 2006. Systematic review: are probiotics useful in controlling gastric colonization by *Helicobacter pylori*? *Aliment Pharmacol Ther* 23 (8):1077–86.

Govindarajan, R., M. Vijayakumar, A. K. Rawat, and S. Mehrotra. 2003. Free radical scavenging potential of Picrorhiza kurrooa Royle ex Benth. *Indian J Exp Biol* 41 (8):875–9.

Grant, H., K. Palmer, R. Riermesma, and M. Oliver. 1989. Duodenal ulcer is associated with low dietary linoleic acid intake. *Gut* 31: 997–998.

Grimes, D. S., and J. Goddard. 1977. Gastric emptying of wholemeal and white bread. *Gut* 18 (9):725–9.

Gupta, A., A. Khajuria, J. Singh, K. L. Bedi, N. K. Satti, P. Dutt, K. A. Suri, O. P. Suri, and G. N. Qazi. 2006. Immunomodulatory activity of biopolymeric fraction RLJ-NE-205 from Picrorhiza kurroa. *Int Immunopharmacol* 6 (10):1543–9.

Ham, M., and J. D. Kaunitz. 2007. Gastroduodenal defense. *Curr Opin Gastroenterol* 23 (6):607–16.

Harris, P.L. et al. 1947. Dietary production of gastric ulcers in rats and prevention by tocopherol administration. *Prod Soc Exp Biol Med* 64.273.

Hidaka, H. et al. 1986. Effects of fructo-oligosaccharides on intestinal flora and human health. *Bifidobacteria Microflora* 5(1):37–50.

Hiraishi, H., T. Sasai, T. Oinuma, T. Shimada, H. Sugaya, and A. Terano. 1999. Polaprezinc protects gastric mucosal cells from noxious agents through antioxidant properties in vitro. *Aliment Pharmacol Ther* 13 (2):261–9.

Hollanders, D., G. Green, I. L. Woolf, B. E. Boyes, R. Y. Wilson, D. J. Cowley, and I. W. Dymock. 1978. Prophylaxis with deglycyrrhizinised liquorice in patients with healed gastric ulcer. *Br Med J* 1 (6106):148.

Hornsby-Lewis, L., M. Shike, P. Brown, M. Klang, D. Pearlstone, and M. F. Brennan. 1994. L-glutamine supplementation in home total parenteral nutrition patients: stability, safety, and effects on intestinal absorption. *JPEN J Parenter Enteral Nutr* 18 (3):268–73.

Huwez, F. U., D. Thirlwell, A. Cockayne, and D. A. Ala'Aldeen. 1998. Mastic gum kills *Helicobacter pylori*. *N Engl J Med* 339 (26):1946.

Ionescu, G. et al. 1990. Oral citrus seed extract in atopic eczema; in vitro and in vivo studies on intestinal microflora. *J Orthomol Med* 5;3:155–158.

Ito, M., T. Tanaka, and Y. Suzuki. 1990. Effect of N-(3-aminopropionyl)-L-histidinato zinc (Z-103) on healing and hydrocortisone-induced relapse of acetic acid ulcers in rats with limited food-intake-time. *Jpn J Pharmacol* 52 (4):513–21.

Ito, M., A. Sato et al. 1998. Mechanism of inhibitory effect of glycyrrhizin on replication of human immunodeficiency virus (HIV). *Antivir Res* 10:289–298.

Jablonska, M. 1995. Healing of gastric body ulcer with gastroprotective versus antisecretory treatment. *Dig Dis Sci* 40 (9):2016–8.

Jarosz, M., J. Dzieniszewski, E. Dabrowska-Ufniarz, M. Wartanowicz, S. Ziemlanski, and P. I. Reed. 1998. Effects of high dose vitamin C treatment on *Helicobacter pylori* infection and total vitamin C concentration in gastric juice. *Eur J Cancer Prev* 7 (6):449–54.

Jaworek, J., T. Brzozowski, and S. J. Konturek. 2005. Melatonin as an organoprotector in the stomach and the pancreas. *J Pineal Res* 38 (2):73–83.

Jones, N. L., S. Shabib, and P. M. Sherman. 1997. Capsaicin as an inhibitor of the growth of the gastric pathogen *Helicobacter pylori*. *FEMS Microbiol Lett* 146 (2):223–7.

Kashimura, H., K. Suzuki, M. Hassan, K. Ikezawa, T. Sawahata, T. Watanabe, A. Nakahara, H. Mutoh, and N. Tanaka. 1999. Polaprezinc, a mucosal protective agent, in combination with lansoprazole, amoxycillin and clarithromycin increases the cure rate of *Helicobacter pylori* infection. *Aliment Pharmacol Ther* 13 (4):483–7.

Kassir, Z. A. 1985. Endoscopic controlled trial of four drug regimens in the treatment of chronic duodenal ulceration. *Ir Med J* 78 (6):153–6.

Kato, K., S. Asai, I. Murai, T. Nagata, Y. Takahashi, S. Komuro, A. Iwasaki, K. Ishikawa, and Y. Arakawa. 2001. Melatonin's gastroprotective and antistress roles involve both central and peripheral effects. *J Gastroenterol* 36 (2):91–5.

Kato, S., H. Nishiwaki, A. Konaka, and K. Takeuchi. 1997. Mucosal ulcerogenic action of monochloramine in rat stomachs: effects of polaprezinc and sucralfate. *Dig Dis Sci* 42 (10):2156–63.

Kato, S., A. Tanaka, Y. Ogawa, K. Kanatsu, K. Seto, T. Yoneda, and K. Takeuchi. 2001. Effect of polaprezinc on impaired healing of chronic gastric ulcers in adjuvant-induced arthritic rats—role of insulin-like growth factors (IGF)-1. *Med Sci Monit* 7 (1):20–5.

Kawamori, T., T. Tanaka, Y. Hirose, M. Ohnishi, and H. Mori. 1996. Inhibitory effects of d-limonene on the development of colonic aberrant crypt foci induced by azoxymethane in F344 rats. *Carcinogenesis* 17 (2):369–72.

Khayyal, M. T., M. Seif-El-Nasr, M. A. El-Ghazaly, S. N. Okpanyi, O. Kelber, and D. Weiser. 2006. Mechanisms involved in the gastro-protective effect of STW 5 (Iberogast) and its components against ulcers and rebound acidity. *Phytomedicine* 13 Suppl 5:56–66.

Khuylusi, S. 1995. The effect of unsaturated fatty acids on *Helicobacter pylori* in vitro. *M Med Micro* 42(4):276–282.

Kim, J. K., S. M. Oh, H. S. Kwon, Y. S. Oh, S. S. Lim, and H. K. Shin. 2006. Anti-inflammatory effect of roasted licorice extracts on lipopolysaccharide-induced inflammatory responses in murine macrophages. *Biochem Biophys Res Commun* 345 (3):1215–23.

Klupinska, G., C. Chojnacki, A. Harasiuk, A. Stepien, P. Wichan, K. Stec-Michalska, and J. Chojnacki. 2006. [Nocturnal secretion of melatonin in subjects with asymptomatic and symptomatic *Helicobacter pylori* infection]. *Pol Merkur Lekarski* 21 (123):239–42.

Klupinska, G., M. Wisniewska-Jarosinska, A. Harasiuk, C. Chojnacki, K. Stec-Michalska, J. Blasiak, R. J. Reiter, and J. Chojnacki. 2006. Nocturnal secretion of melatonin in patients with upper digestive tract disorders. *J Physiol Pharmacol* 57 Suppl 5:41–50.

Kohli, Y., Y. Suto, and T. Kodama. 1981. Effect of hypoxia on acetic acid ulcer of the stomach in rats with or without coenzyme Q10. *Jpn J Exp Med* 51 (2):105–8.

Komarov, F. I., S. I. Rappoport, N. K. Malinovskaia, L. A. Voznesenskaia, and L. Vetterberg. 2003. [Melatonin: ulcer disease and seasons of the year]. *Klin Med* (Mosk) 81 (9):17–21.

Konturek, S. J., P. C. Konturek, I. Brzozowska, M. Pawlik, Z. Sliwowski, M. Czesnikiewicz-Guzik, S. Kwiecien, T. Brzozowski, G. A. Bubenik, and W. W. Pawlik. 2007. Localization and biological activities of melatonin in intact and diseased gastrointestinal tract (GIT). *J Physiol Pharmacol* 58 (3):381–405.

Konturek, S. J., P. C. Konturek, and T. Brzozowski. 2005. Prostaglandins and ulcer healing. *J Physiol Pharmacol* 56 Suppl 5:5–31.

Kositchaiwat, C., S. Kositchaiwat, and J. Havanondha. 1993. Curcuma longa Linn. in the treatment of gastric ulcer comparison to liquid antacid: a controlled clinical trial. *J Med Assoc Thai* 76 (11):601–5.

Krajci, W. M., and D. L. Lynch. 1997. The inhibition of various microorganisms, by crude walnut hulls and juglone. *Microbios Letters* 4:175–181.

Krausse, R., J. Bielenberg, W. Blaschek, and U. Ullmann. 2004. In vitro anti-*Helicobacter pylori* activity of Extractum liquiritiae, glycyrrhizin and its metabolites. *J Antimicrob Chemother* 54 (1):243–6.

Langmead, L., and D. S. Rampton. 2001. Review article: herbal treatment in gastrointestinal and liver disease—benefits and dangers. *Aliment Pharmacol Ther* 15 (9):1239–52.

Larkworthy, W., and P. F. Holgate. 1975. Deglycyrrhizinized liquorice in the treatment of chronic duodenal ulcer. A retrospective endoscopic survey of 32 patients. *Practitioner* 215 (1290):787–92.

Larkworthy, W., P. F. Holgate, M. B. McIllmurray, and M. J. Langman. 1977. Deglycyrrhizinised liquorice in duodenal ulcer. *Br Med J* 2 (6095):1123.

Lesbros-Pantoflickova, D., I. Corthesy-Theulaz, and A. L. Blum. 2007. *Helicobacter pylori* and probiotics. *J Nutr* 137 (3 Suppl 2):812S–8S.

Lin, Y. T., Y. I. Kwon, R. G. Labbe, and K. Shetty. 2005. Inhibition of *Helicobacter pylori* and associated urease by oregano and cranberry phytochemical synergies. *Appl Environ Microbiol* 71 (12):8558–64.

Lindenbaum, E. S., and J. J. Mueller. 1974. Effects of pyridoxine on mice after immobilization stress. *Nutr Metab* 17 (6):368–74.

Mahmood, A., A. J. FitzGerald, T. Marchbank, E. Ntatsaki, D. Murray, S. Ghosh, and R. J. Playford. 2007. Zinc carnosine, a health food supplement that stabilises small bowel integrity and stimulates gut repair processes. *Gut* 56 (2):168–75.

Malhotra, S. L. 1978. A comparison of unrefined wheat and rice diets in the management of duodenal ulcer. *Postgrad Med J* 54 (627):6–9.

Malinovskaia, N. K., F. I. Komarova, S. I. Rapoport, N. T. Raikhlin, I. M. Kvetnoi, A. A. Lakshin, L. A. Voznesenskaia, and M. I. Rasulov. 2006. [Melatonin in treatment of duodenal ulcer]. *Klin Med* (Mosk) 84 (1):5–11.

Malinovskaia, N. K., S. I. Rapoport, N. I. Zhernakova, S. N. Rybnikova, L. I. Postnikova, and I. E. Parkhomenko. 2007. [Antihelicobacter effects of melatonin]. *Klin Med* (Mosk) 85 (3):40–3.

Malinovskaya, N., F. I. Komarov, S. I. Rapoport, L. A. Voznesenskaya, and L. Wetterberg. 2001. Melatonin production in patients with duodenal ulcer. *Neuro Endocrinol Lett* 22 (2):109–17.

Matsukura, T., and H. Tanaka. 2000. Applicability of zinc complex of L-carnosine for medical use. *Biochemistry* (Mosc) 65 (7):817–23.

McKellar, R. C. et al. 1989. Metabolism of fructo-oligosaccharides by Bifidobacterium spp. *App Microbiol Biotechnol* 31:537–541.

Moorehead, L. 1915. Contributions to the physiology of the stomach. XXVIII. Further studies on the action of the bitter tonic on the secretion of gastric juice. *J Pharmacol Exper Therap* 7:577–589.

Morgan, R. J. et al. 1982. The effect of deglycyrrhizinized liquorice on the occurrence of aspirin and aspirin plus bile acid-induced gastric lesions, and aspirin absorption in rats. *Gastroenterology* 82:1134.

Morris, T. J., B. J. Calcraft, J. Rhodes, D. Hole, and M. S. Morton. 1974. Effect of a deglycyrrhizinised liquorice compound on the gastric mucosal barrier of the dog. *Digestion* 11 (5–6):355–63.

Multicentre Trial. 1973. Treatment of duodenal ulcer with glycyrrhizinic-acid-reduced liquorice. *Brit Med J* 773(3):501–504.

Murray, M. T. *Natural Alternatives to Over-the-counter and Prescription Drugs* (New York: William Morrow, 1994).

Nakaizumi, A., M. Baba, H. Uehara, H. Iishi, and M. Tatsuta. 1997. d-Limonene inhibits N-nitrosobis(2-

oxopropyl)amine induced hamster pancreatic carcinogenesis. *Cancer Lett* 117 (1):99–103.

Nishiwaki, H., S. Kato, S. Sugamoto, M. Umeda, H. Morita, T. Yoneta, and K. Takeuchi. 1999. Ulcerogenic and healing impairing actions of monochloramine in rat stomachs: effects of zinc L-carnosine, polaprezinc. *J Physiol Pharmacol* 50 (2):183–95.

Okabe, S., K. Honda, K. Takeuchi, and K. Takagi. 1975. Inhibitory effect of L-glutamine on gastric irritation and back diffusion of gastric acid in response to aspirin in the rat. *Am J Dig Dis* 20 (7):626–31.

Olukoga, A., and D. Donaldson. 2000. Liquorice and its health implications. *J R Soc Health* 120 (2):83–9.

O'Mahony, R., H. Al-Khtheeri, D. Weerasekera, N. Fernando, D. Vaira, J. Holton, and C. Basset. 2005. Bactericidal and anti-adhesive properties of culinary and medicinal plants against *Helicobacter pylori*. World *J Gastroenterol* 11 (47):7499–507.

Oner, G., N. M. Bor, E. Onuk, and Z. N. Oner. 1981. The role of zinc ion in the development of gastric ulcers in rats. *Eur J Pharmacol* 70 (2):241–3.

Osadchuk, M. A., and AIu Kulidzhanov. 2005. [Melanin-producing and NO-synthase gastric cells and the processes of cell regeneration in gastric and duodenal ulcers]. *Klin Med* (Mosk) 83 (9):34–7.

Pereira Rde, S. 2006. Regression of gastroesophageal reflux disease symptoms using dietary supplementation with melatonin, vitamins and aminoacids: comparison with omeprazole. *J Pineal Res* 41 (3):195–200.

Petry, J. J., and S. K. Hadley. 2001. Medicinal herbs: answers and advice, Part 2. *Hosp Pract* (Minneap) 36 (8):55–9.

Pompei, R., O. Flore, M. A. Marccialis, A. Pani, and B. Loddo. 1979. Glycyrrhizic acid inhibits virus growth and inactivates virus particles. *Nature* 281 (5733):689–90.

Puri, A., R. P. Saxena, P. Y. Guru, D. K. Kulshreshtha, K. C. Saxena, and B. N. Dhawan. 1992. Immunostimulant Activity of Picroliv, the Iridoid Glycoside Fraction of Picrorhiza kurroa, and its Protective Action against Leishmania donovani Infection in Hamsters1. *Planta Med* 58 (6):528–32.

Rafatullah, S., M. Tariq, M. A. Al-Yahya, J. S. Mossa, and A. M. Ageel. 1990. Evaluation of turmeric (Curcuma longa) for gastric and duodenal antiulcer activity in rats. *J Ethnopharmacol* 29 (1):25–34.

Rapoport, S. I., N. T. Raikhlin, N. K. Malinovskaia, and A. A. Lakshin. 2003. [Ultrastructural changes in cells of the antral gastric mucosa in patients with duodenal ulcers treated with melatonin]. *Ter Arkh* 75 (2):10–4.

Rappaport, E. M. 1955. Achlorhydria; associated symptoms and response to hydrochloric acid. *N Engl J Med* 252 (19):802–5.

Rasche, R., and W. C. Butterfield. 1973. Vitamin A pretreatment of stress ulcers in rats. *Arch Surg* 106 (3):320–1.

Rees, W. D., J. Rhodes, J. E. Wright, L. F. Stamford, and A. Bennett. 1979. Effect of deglycyrrhizinated liquorice on gastric mucosal damage by aspirin. *Scand J Gastroenterol* 14 (5):605–7.

———. 1979. Effect of deglycyrrhizinated liquorice on gastric mucosal damage by aspirin. *Scand J Gastroenterol* 14 (5):605–7.

Reiter, R. J., D. X. Tan, J. C. Mayo, R. M. Sainz, J. Leon, and D. Bandyopadhyay. 2003. Neurally-mediated and neurally-independent beneficial actions of melatonin in the gastrointestinal tract. *J Physiol Pharmacol* 54 Suppl 4:113–25.

Rodriguez de la, S.A., and M. az-Rubio. 1994. Multicenter clinical trial of zinc acexamate in the prevention of nonsteroidal antiinflammatory drug induced gastroenteropathy. Spanish Study Group on NSAID Induced Gastroenteropathy Prevention. *J Rheumatol* 21(5):927–33.

Romero, C., E. Medina, J. Vargas, M. Brenes, and A. De Castro. 2007. In vitro activity of olive oil polyphenols against *Helicobacter pylori*. *J Agric Food Chem* 55 (3):680–6.

Russell, R. I., J. E. N. Dickie. 1968. Clinical trial of a deglycyrrhizinized liquorice preparation in peptic ulcer. *J Ther Clin Res* 2:2.

Russell, R. I., R. J. Morgan, and L. M. Nelson. 1984. Studies on the protective effect of deglycyrrhinised liquorice against aspirin (ASA) and ASA plus bile acid-induced gastric mucosal damage, and ASA absorption in rats. *Scand J Gastroenterol* Suppl 92:97–100.

Rydning, A., A. Berstad, E. Aadland, and B. Odegaard. 1982. Prophylactic effect of dietary fibre in duodenal ulcer disease. *Lancet* 2 (8301):736–9.

Satyanarayana, M. N. 2006. Capsaicin and gastric ulcers. *Crit Rev Food Sci Nutr* 46 (4):275–328.

Seiki, M., S. Ueki, Y. Tanaka, M. Soeda, Y. Hori, H. Aita, T. Yoneta, H. Morita, E. Tagashira, and S. Okabe. 1990. [Studies on anti-ulcer effects of a new compound, zinc L-carnosine (Z-103)]. *Nippon Yakurigaku Zasshi* 95 (5):257–69.

Sempertegui, F., M. Diaz, R. Mejia, O. G. Rodriguez-Mora, E. Renteria, C. Guarderas, B. Estrella, R. Recalde, D. H. Hamer, and P. G. Reeves. 2007. Low concentrations of zinc in gastric mucosa are associated with increased severity of *Helicobacter pylori*-induced inflammation. *Helicobacter* 12 (1):43–8.

Sener, G., F. O. Goren, N. B. Ulusoy, Y. Ersoy, S. Arbak, and G. A. Dulger. 2005. Protective effect of melatonin and omeprazole against alendronat-induced gastric damage. *Dig Dis Sci* 50 (8):1506–12.

Sharma, M. L., C. S. Rao, and P. L. Duda. 1994. Immunostimulatory activity of Picrorhiza kurroa leaf extract. *J Ethnopharmacol* 41 (3):185–92.

Shimada, T., N. Watanabe, Y. Ohtsuka, M. Endoh, K. Kojima, H. Hiraishi, and A. Terano. 1999. Polaprezinc down-regulates proinflammatory cytokine-induced nuclear factor-kappaB activiation and interleukin-8 expression in gastric epithelial cells. *J Pharmacol Exp Ther* 291 (1):345–52.

Shive, W., R. N. Snider, B. Dubilier, J. C. Rude, G. E. Clark, Jr., and J. O. Ravel. 1957. Glutamine in treatment of peptic ulcer; preliminary report. *Tex State J Med* 53 (11):840–2.

Shmuely, H., J. Yahav, Z. Samra, G. Chodick, R. Koren, Y. Niv, and I. Ofek. 2007. Effect of cranberry juice on eradication of *Helicobacter pylori* in patients treated with antibiotics and a proton pump inhibitor. *Mol Nutr Food Res* 51 (6):746–51.

Sikka, K. K. et al. 1988. Efficacy of dried raw banana powder in the healing of peptic ulcer. *J Assoc Physicians India* 36:65–66.

Singh, P., V. K. Bhargava, and S. K. Garg. 2002. Effect of melatonin and beta-carotene on indomethacin induced gastric mucosal injury. *Indian J Physiol Pharmacol* 46 (2):229–34.

Smit, H. F., B. H. Kroes, A. J. van den Berg, D. van der Wal, E. van den Worm, C. J. Beukelman, H. van Dijk, and R. P. Labadie. 2000. Immunomodulatory and anti-inflammatory activity of Picrorhiza scrophulariiflora. *J Ethnopharmacol* 73 (1–2):101–9.

Souba, W. W., V. S. Klimberg, R. D. Hautamaki, W. H. Mendenhall, F. C. Bova, R. J. Howard, K. I. Bland, and E. M. Copeland. 1990. Oral glutamine reduces bacterial translocation following abdominal radiation. *J Surg Res* 48 (1):1–5.

Spaeth, G., R. D. Berg, R. D. Specian, and E. A. Deitch. 1990. Food without fiber promotes bacterial translocation from the gut. *Surgery* 108 (2):240–6; discussion 246–7.

Stenson, W. F., D. Cort, J. Rodgers, R. Burakoff, K. DeSchryver-Kecskemeti, T. L. Gramlich, and W. Beeken. 1992. Dietary supplementation with fish oil in ulcerative colitis. *Ann Intern Med* 116 (8):609–14.

Sun, M., H. W. Fan, H. Y. Ma, and Q. Zhu. 2007. [Protective effect of total glucosides of Picrorhiza scrophulariiflora against oxidative stress in glomerular mesangial cells induced by high glucose]. *Yao Xue Xue Bao* 42 (4):381–5.

Suzuki, H., M. Mori, K. Seto, M. Miyazawa, A. Kai, M. Suematsu, T. Yoneta, S. Miura, and H. Ishii. 2001. Polaprezinc attenuates the *Helicobacter pylori*-induced gastric mucosal leucocyte activation in Mongolian gerbils—a study using intravital video-microscopy. *Aliment Pharmacol Ther* 15 (5):715–25.

Suzuki, H., M. Mori, K. Seto, S. Nagahashi, C. Kawaguchi, H. Morita, M. Suzuki, S. Miura, T. Yoneta, and H. Ishii. 1999. Polaprezinc, a gastroprotective agent: attenuation of monochloramine-evoked gastric DNA fragmentation. *J Gastroenterol* 34 Suppl 11:43–6.

Tewari, S. N., and A. K. Wilson. 1972. Deglycyrrhizinated liquorice in duodenal ulcer. *Practitioner* 210:820.

Thamlikitkul, V., N. Bunyapraphatsara, T. Dechatiwongse, S. Theerapong, C. Chantrakul, T. Thanaveerasuwan, S. Nimitnon, P. Boonroj, W. Punkrut, V. Gingsungneon et al. 1989. Randomized double blind study of Curcuma domestica Val. for dyspepsia. *J Med Assoc Thai* 72 (11):613–20.

Thomas, M., J. Sheran, N. Smith, S. Fonseca, and A. J. Lee. 2007. AKL1, a botanical mixture for the treatment of asthma: a randomised, double-blind, placebo-controlled, cross-over study. *BMC Pulm Med* 7:4.

Tran, C. D., M. A. Campbell, Y. Kolev, S. Chamberlain, H. Q. Huynh, and R. N. Butler. 2005. Short-term zinc supplementation attenuates Helicobacter felis-induced gastritis in the mouse. *J Infect* 50 (5):417–24.

Turcan, M., A. Iacobovici, and I. Haulica. 1997. [Melatonin and ubiquinone as endogenous antioxidant factors]. *Rev Med Chir Soc Med Nat Iasi* 101 (1–2):92–7.

Turpie, A. G., J. Runcie, and T. J. Thomson. 1969. Clinical trial of deglydyrrhizinized liquorice in gastric ulcer. *Gut* 10 (4):299–302.

Uedo, N., M. Tatsuta, H. Iishi, M. Baba, N. Sakai, H. Yano, and T. Otani. 1999. Inhibition by D-limonene of gastric carcinogenesis induced by N-methyl-N'-nitro-N-nitrosoguanidine in Wistar rats. *Cancer Lett* 137 (2):131–6.

Vaidya, A. B., D. S. Antarkar, J. C. Doshi, A. D. Bhatt, V. Ramesh, P. V. Vora, D. Perissond, A. J. Baxi, and P. M. Kale. 1996. Picrorhiza kurroa (Kutaki) Royle ex Benth as a hepatoprotective agent—experimental & clinical studies. *J Postgrad Med* 42 (4):105–8.

van der Hulst, R. R., B. K. van Kreel, M. F. von Meyenfeldt, R. J. Brummer, J. W. Arends, N. E. Deutz, and P. B. Soeters. 1993. Glutamine and the preservation of gut integrity. *Lancet* 341 (8857):1363–5.

van Marle, J. et al. 1981. Deglycyrrhizinised liquorice (DGL) and the renewal of rat stomach epithelium. *Eur J Pharmcol* 72:219–225.

Varas, Lorenzo, M. J., M. A. Lopez, B. J. Gordillo, and S. J. Mundet. 1991. Comparative study of 3 drugs (aceglutamide aluminum, zinc acexamate, and magaldrate) in the long-term maintenance treatment (1 year) of peptic ulcer. *Rev Esp Enferm Dig* 80(2):91–4.

Vargha, G., and F. Damrau. 1963. Standardized cabbage factor complex for peptic ulcers. Report of animal experiments and 162 ambulatory cases. *J Am Med Womens Assoc* 18:460–3.

Vattem, D. A., R. Ghaedian, and K. Shetty. 2005. Enhancing health benefits of berries through phenolic antioxidant enrichment: focus on cranberry. *Asia Pac J Clin Nutr* 14 (2):120–30.

Watanabe, S., X. E. Wang, M. Hirose, T. Kivilioto, T. Osada, H. Miwa, H. Oide, T. Kitamura, T. Yoneta, K. Seto, and N. Sato. 1998. Insulin-like growth factor I plays a role in gastric wound healing: evidence using a zinc derivative, polaprezinc, and an in vitro rabbit wound repair model. *Aliment Pharmacol Ther* 12 (11):1131–8.

Webb, P. M., C. J. Bates, D. Palli, and D. Forman. 1997. Gastric cancer, gastritis and plasma vitamin C: results from an international correlation and cross-sectional study. The Eurogast Study Group. *Int J Cancer* 73 (5):684–9.

Werbach, M. R. 2008. Melatonin for the treatment of gastroesophageal reflux disease. *Altern Ther Health Med* 14 (4):54–8.

Willette, R. C., L. Barrow, R. Doster, J. Wilkins, J. S. Wilkins, and J. P. Heggers. Purified d-limonene: an effective agent for the relief of occasional symptoms of heartburn. Proprietary study. WRC Laboratories, Inc. Galveston, TX.

Wright, J., and A. Gaby. *The Patient's Book of Natural Healing*. Rocklin (Rocklin, CA: Prima Publishing Co., 1999).

Yano, H., M. Tatsuta, H. Iishi, M. Baba, N. Sakai, and N. Uedo. 1999. Attenuation by d-limonene of sodium chloride-enhanced gastric carcinogenesis induced by N-methyl-N'-nitro-N-nitrosoguanidine in Wistar rats. *Int J Cancer* 82 (5):665–8.

Yoshikawa, M., Y. Matsui, H. Kawamoto, N. Umemoto, K. Oku, M. Koizumi, J. Yamao, S. Kuriyama, H. Nakano, N. Hozumi, S. Ishizaka, and H. Fukui. 1997. Effects of glycyrrhizin on immune-mediated cyto-toxicity. *J Gastroenterol Hepatol* 12 (3):243–8.

Yoshikawa, T., Y. Naito, T. Tanigawa, T. Yoneta, M. Yasuda, S. Ueda, H. Oyamada, and M. Kondo. 1991. Effect of zinc-carnosine chelate compound (Z-103), a novel antioxidant, on acute gastric mucosal injury induced by ischemia-reperfusion in rats. *Free Radic Res Commun* 14 (4):289–96.

Zhang, H. M., N. Wakisaka, O. Maeda, and T. Yama-moto. 1997. Vitamin C inhibits the growth of a bacterial risk factor for gastric carcinoma: *Helicobacter pylori*. *Cancer* 80 (10):1897–903.

Zhang, L., J. Ma, K. Pan, V. L. Go, J. Chen, and W. C. You. 2005. Efficacy of cranberry juice on *Helicobacter pylori* infection: a double-blind, randomized placebo-controlled trial. *Helicobacter* 10 (2):139–45.

Zhang, Y., D. L. DeWitt, S. Murugesan, and M. G. Nair. 2004. Novel lipid-peroxidation- and cyclooxygenase-inhibitory tannins from Picrorhiza kurroa seeds. *Chem Biodivers* 1 (3):426–41.

Zhang, Y., D. L. Dewitt, S. Murugesan, and M. G. Nair. 2005. Cyclooxygenase-2 enzyme inhibitory triterpenoids from Picrorhiza kurroa seeds. *Life Sci* 77 (25):3222–30.

Ziegler, T. R., K. Benfell, R. J. Smith, L. S. Young, E. Brown, E. Ferrari-Baliviera, D. K. Lowe, and D. W.

Wilmore. 1990. Safety and metabolic effects of L-glutamine administration in humans. *JPEN J Parenter Enteral Nutr* 14 (4 Suppl):137S–146S.

Zullo, A., V. Rinaldi, C. Hassan, F. Diana, S. Winn, G. Castagna, and A. F. Attili. 2000. Ascorbic acid and intestinal metaplasia in the stomach: a prospective, randomized study. *Aliment Pharmacol Ther* 14 (10):1303–9.

Pharmaceutical Companies
Industry Size

AstraZeneca. Annual Report 2006. http://www .astrazeneca.com/sites/7/imagebank/type Articleparam511715/astrazeneca-annual-report-20F-2006.pdf (accessed January 10, 2008).

Latner, A. 2000. The top 200 drugs of 1999. *Pharmacy Times* 66:16–33.

Visiongain. *Gastrointestinal Disorders Market Intelligence to 2012*. May 25, 2007.

Pharmaceutical Companies
Conflicts of Interest

Angell, M. 2000. Is academic medicine for sale? *N Engl J Med* 342 (20):1516–8.

———. 2000. The pharmaceutical industry—to whom is it accountable? *N Engl J Med* 342 (25):1902–4.

Boyd, E. A., and L. A. Bero. 2000. Assessing faculty financial relationships with industry: A case study. *JAMA* 284 (17):2209–14.

Center for Public Integrity. Drug Lobby Second to None: How the Pharmaceutical Industry Gets Its Way in Washington. http://www.publicintegrity.org/rx/report.aspx?aid=723 (accessed March 20, 2008).

Center for Science in the Public Interest. Conflicts of Interest on Cox-2 Panel. http://www.cspinet.org/new/200502251.html (accessed January 28, 2008).

Cho, M. K., R. Shohara, A. Schissel, and D. Rennie. 2000. Policies on faculty conflicts of interest at US universities. *JAMA* 284 (17):2203–8.

Rubin R., FDA Called "Cozy" with Drugmakers USA Today. http://www.usatoday.com/news/health/2007-06-11-fda-drugmakers_N.htm?csp=34&POE=click-refer (accessed March 20, 2008).

Schmit, J., Bush Budget Plan's Drug Fees Attacked *USA Today*, February 14, 2007. http://www.usatoday.com/money/industries/health/drugs/2007-02-14-fda-budget-usat_x.html (accessed January 28, 2008).

Food and Drug Administration Amendments Act of 2007. http://www.fda.gov/oc/initiatives/HR3580.pdf (accessed January 28, 2008).

Reference Articles

Andres, M. R., Jr., and J. R. Bingham. 1970. Tubeless gastric analysis with a radiotelemetering pill (Heidelberg capsule). *Can Med Assoc J* 102 (10):1087–9.

Clermont College, University of Cincinnati. Digestive System. http://biology.clc.uc.edu/courses/bio105/digestiv.html and http://biology.clc.uc.edu/courses/bio115/pepsin.html (accessed March 27, 2008).

Dressman, J. B., R. R. Berardi, L. C. Dermentzoglou, T. L. Russell, S. P. Schmaltz, J. L. Barnett, and K. M. Jarvenpaa. 1990. Upper gastrointestinal (GI) pH in young, healthy men and women. *Pharm Res* 7 (7):756–61.

Fries, J. F. 1992. Assessing and understanding patient risk. Scand *J Rheumatol* Suppl 92:21–4.

Rogers, S. A. *No More Heartburn: Stop the Pain in 30 Days—Naturally!: The Safe, Effective Way to Prevent and Heal Chronic Gastrointestinal Disorders* (New York: Kensington Books, 2000).

Wikipedia contributors, Stomach, *Wikipedia, The Free Encyclopedia*, http://en.wikipedia.org/w/index.php ?title=Stomach&oldid=258470505 (accessed January 6, 2008).

Wright J., and L. Lenard. *Why Stomach Acid Is Good For You: Natural Relief For Heartburn, Indigestion, and GERD* (New York: M Evans & Company, Inc., 2001).

Index